My (Our) Chance for a Change in Spite of My (Our) Obstacles

Gulf Coast and White House Included

By

Dorothy R. Francis

Bloomington, IN 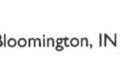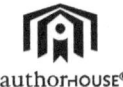 Milton Keynes, UK

authorHOUSE®

AuthorHouse™
1663 Liberty Drive, Suite 200
Bloomington, IN 47403
www.authorhouse.com
Phone: 1-800-839-8640

AuthorHouse™ UK Ltd.
500 Avebury Boulevard
Central Milton Keynes, MK9 2BE
www.authorhouse.co.uk
Phone: 08001974150

First published by AuthorHouse 11/25/2008

ISBN: 978-1-4259-9299-6 (sc)

Printed in the United States of America
Bloomington, Indiana

This book is printed on acid-free paper.

Dear Readers,

For years I have attempted to put these words on paper and haven't been able to until Karen had died (cancer); until my darling daughter Lisa had died (suicide) from the curse.

Curses has been in our lives since the beginning of time. Adam was under a curse when he let Eve cohort him into eating of the fruit. Eve was under a curse when she listen to the Devil. The Devil was under a curse when he convince Eve that she could eat of the tree and not die; her eyes would be opened and she would be like God knowing good and evil.

We were born under a curse because of Adam. We were born under a curse because of generation past. The curse (Sin) I am now speaking of is the choices we are making now as a society. The curses I am now speaking of is how we are making our children stumble. The curse I am speaking of now is neglect, abuses, abandonment, depression, repression, murder, addiction, etc. and because we are under so much weight and can't seem to get back on top we are sinning and committing all sources of things which are against God. The world is in a corrupt state and getting worse, and as long as the world is corrupt, we are all going to be cursed.

Bishop Noel Jones speaks of how sin is transferred from one to another as a money or wire transfer. Father Paul McQuillen speaks of how we as a society must be less tolerant of what others do and say because we all are going to be held accountable for our actions.

Pastor Paula White and Pastor Larry Huch speaks about the releasing of the Generational Blessing and Breaking from the Curse (Repression- Depression). Bishop T.D. Jakes speaks about how we can be Liberated from all of the bondage.

Christ broke the curse thought death. He redeemed us from the curse of the law by becoming a curse for us, for it is written:" Cursed is everyone who is hung on the tree." He redeemed us in order that the blessing given to Abraham might come to the Gentiles through Christ Jesus, so that by faith we might receive the promise of the Spirit." Galatians 3:13-14; For we were called to be free, but we are not to use our freedom to indulge the sinful nature; rather serve one another in love. The entire law is summed up in a single command: Love our neighbor as ourselves." If we keep on biting and devouring each other, watch out and we will be destroyed by each other." Galatians 5:13-15

To my readers, I really believe that the curse can be broken if we heed to the words of God (Jesus). The Lord sends Blessings and Curses. The Blessings if we obey the commands of the Lord our God and a Curse if we disobey the commands of the Lord our God and turn from the way that He command us today by following other gods, which we have not known" Deuteronomy 11: 26-28

Dorothy R. Francis:

Dedicated to:

My daughter who I fought hard for and lost (Lisa)

Lorisa
Deidra
Derika
De'niche
Harold
Keone
Isaiah

All of my foster children

Also a special thanks to: St. Joseph The Worker Catholic Church- (Marrero La.) Fr. Paul McQuillen;

Blessed be the Holy Name of Jesus- (Los Angeles Ca.) Fr. Paul and Fr. Joseph; St Philip the Apostle

Catholic Church and Westside Baptist Church- (Lewisville Texas) Bishop Blakes

Dr. Candice Cutrone- (Psychiatry)— Mental Health (Algier branch- Dr. Wantpa)—Family Service of

Greater New Orleans (Gretna branch-Ginger and Lydia)— Y.W.C.A. (Gretna and Slidell branch).

Y.W.C.A. (Compton branch-Cynthia)—Southern Christian Leadership Conference of Greater Los Angeles

(Rosa Parks A.S.C.C.—Aggy and Stephanie)—West Jefferson Medical Center (Marrero La.)—Oschner

Foundation Hospital (Jefferson Highway)

Karen, my cousin, sister, friend has slipped away. Karen my cousin, sister, friend has passed away. Karen my dear cousin has now moved on. The reality of Karen's death has now set in. The reality that there will be no more calls to Karen to see how she is doing has now set in. The reality that there will be no more calls to Karen to tell her that I love her has now set in. The reality has really set in now that Karen my beloved cousin has now gone on.

Karen was in her forty's when she died. Karen was in her forty's with a terrible illness (cancer) that eventually killed her.

The Saturday after Karen had died, Celtic, Boss (my daughter's dogs) and myself are home alone. We are home alone and I am down and out thinking about how life is so unfair, and how it is taking the children faster than the parents.

I am so engrossed in my thinking (thoughts) that suddenly tears starts to flow from my eyes and there is no one shoulder to lay my head on. I am so engrossed in my thoughts and tears and there is no one's shoulder to cry on. I am so engrossed in my thoughts and tears and there is no one to talk to, to tell them how and what I am feeling, and just as the tears begins to fall; and just as the thunder begins to roll; and just as the lightening begins to flash, my daughter's dog (Celtic) jumps on the sofa (couch) and puts his paws on my back as if he is trying to tell me that everything is going to be alright. As if to tell me that everything is going to be alright (well) in my soul.

Saturday has now come again. It is the day of Karen's funeral and Celtic, Boss and I are home alone again. The clock is ticking (moving) toward eight (8) AM California's time, ten ((10) AM Louisiana time, and I am thinking about Karen's Funeral, and Karen's life, when suddenly I began to mediate on Jesus the Healer and how he heals all our aches and pains. I am sitting and meditating on Jesus and I remember (realize) that I have no control over what was happening to Karen, because what was happening to me (my children), because what was happening to her was God's will and not man's will.

I decided that maybe I needed to have a little talk with Jesus; to tell Him all about our troubles. He would hear our feeble cry and answer by and by. I'll feel a little prayer wheel turning and I'll know there's fire burning, I needed to have a little talk with Jesus to make things right.

So I started talking to Jesus. I started telling Him all about our troubles. I started thanking Him for all that he had done for Karen. I started thanking Him for all He had done for me (my children). I started telling Him that no matter what happens from that moment on, I would keep on praising Him; keep on praising His name.

Just as I am telling Jesus that no matter what happens from that moment on, I would keep on praising His name; I looked up and saw Celtic falling. I looked up and saw Celtic falling and shaking trying to stand up. I didn't fully comprehend what was happening to him, because I was in the company of Jesus having a little talk with Him. I didn't fully comprehend what was happening to him because I was deep in prayer.

I jump up and went to Celtic. He was limped; He was shaking, and his mouth was wet from his spitting up. I suddenly realized that Celtic my pal; Celtic my buddy; Celtic my friend was in a crisis (trouble). I suddenly realized that he was having a Seizure.

At first I didn't know what to do. At first I was frighten (anxious) and almost out of control. At first I thought he was going to die. In thinking that possibly he was going to die, I then realized that I needed to compose myself and do what ever it took to try to get my friend through what he was going through.

I then tried to get him to relax. I then tried to get me to relax. I then started rubbing his back. I then started rubbing his back, calling his name and telling him everything was going to be alright. The more I rubbed his back, the more he seemed to get limp. I started rubbing him on the back, stomach, and started adding prayers to the mix. I started rubbing, praying all at the same time. The limber he got, the more I prayed, the more I prayed, the limber he got. I then prayed a heart wrenching prayer. I prayed from my heart. I prayed from my soul, and just as suddenly as I prayed and cried from my soul, I remembered that I had just told Jesus (God) that no matter what happens in my life from that moment on, I would keep on praising His name.

Upon remembering the promise, upon remembering the conversation I had just had with Jesus (God); I thought about the Lord's Prayer; I thought about God's will, and not man's will. I then thought about how no matter what had happened to Karen; no matter what had happened to me; no matter what had happened to my children (grandchildren); no matter what had happened to Celtic (Boss) would be the will of God, a will that I have no control over; a will I need only to accept, because the only control I have in life is to obey God.

I started rubbing Celtic back (stomach). I started trying to extend to him the same courtesy, love, kindness and support that he had tried to give me. I tried to give him back the time and attention he had given me that not many humans had given. I tried to extend the kindness that Karen my cousin had given me.

Karen was a younger cousin who had been adopted by my uncle who had married her mom, and like so many marriages; when the marriage falls apart, the relationship with the children falls apart also.

After the breakup of the marriage, Karen's mom, Karen and I would run into each other from time to time. Whenever I would run into them, they would still treat me as before. They would treat me as niece, cousin; and I would treat them as auntie, cousin and friend. Our relationship stayed the same.

My heart aches for Karen. My heart aches for Karen because I know how she ached for her adopted father. My heart aches for Karen because I know how she ached for a hug (word) from her adopted father as she had from her biological (Heavenly) father. A hug from her adopted father even though the bond had been broken so many years before.

Karen has gone on to her Heavenly Father and I am left behind yearning for a hug from my earthly (biological) father. A hug from my father whose care I was placed in many years before. This bond has been broken also. This bond has been broken and I have now fallen down and have been made naked.

I forgot about the times I got up dressed. I forgot about the times I fell down, had struggles; had tribulations; had pain, and was picked up by my Heavenly Father.

I forgot about the unlimited amount of power and resources my Father has. I forgot about the goodness of my Father and how His mercy endures forever. I forgot about the countless times He redeemed me from the hands of my enemies and made my enemies my foot stool. I forgot how He gathered me from the East and the West; from the North and the South, and how I wandered in the Wilderness in a solitary way and found no city to dwell in. I forgot how hungry and thirsty I was and how my soul fainted (like Jesus in the desert). I just forgot what my Father did altogether.

There is a reason I am looking for my Father now. The reason I am looking for my Father now is because I have been made a prisoner. The reason I am looking for my Father now is because I am in a prison cell.

I have been in a prison cell previously and My Father has had me released. I took my Father for granted upon my releases and just assumed that He was going to bail me out as before.

I feel this time is different. I feel as though this time there is not going to be a release. I feel this time is different because my jailer has locked the doors to my prison cell and has thrown away the key. The Prosecutor is no different, the Prosecutor feels that I have beat the system too many time previously. This time he has gained new evidence that can keep me locked up for a very long time. I now feel the pain of being thrown in prison. I now feel the pain of being broken; downhearted; shaken, feeling as though I am all alone and at the end of my rope, needing to put an end to my misery so that I wouldn't have to go through this agony again. I failed to recall that my Father (God) is my rescuer, I failed to recall that God is my strength; I failed to recall that if I go to Him in the right way that He would respond to my pain and suffering and have me released.

In my misery, I forgot that St. Paul said," the suffering and trials of the present are destined to be only a prelude to the glorious future of the children of God. To consider the suffering of the present time nothing compared with the glory to be revealed to us. For creation was made subjection of the futility; not of its own occur, but because of the one subjected to it, in hope that creation itself is groaning in labor pains until now; and not just that, but we ourselves who have the first fruit of the Spirit, we also groan with ourselves as we wait for the adoption, and the redemption of our body." Roman 8:18-23 Holy Bible

I am not free. I feel as though I am in a dream. I feel as though I am in a trance, wondering when this nightmare is going to end. I feel the only option I have; the only recourse I have is to end this nightmare; is to end this insanity, so as not to endure this pain, suffering and bondage again.

I feel this way because I have not exited jail. I feel this way because there is no peace. I feel this way because there is no joy. I feel this way because there has never been an ounce of permanence in my life. The only permanence I seem to have had has been when they locked me up and thrown away the key. The only permanence I ever had has been when they locked me up; thrown away the key, and made me naked.

Samson, the strongest man of his generation knew the hardship of prison. He also felt that he had to end his pain and suffering (imprisonment). Samson's suffering and pain was brought about because of the flesh. His suffering was brought on because he was unable to control his lust for unattainable women. In his lust for the unattainable, he disobeyed God, his parents, and anyone else who stool in his way. He married an evil Philistine woman (Delilah) who brought him down to his knees and robbed him of his might.

Samson was no ordinary man. He was born to a special class of people (Jesus-David- Nazarene) who were devout people of God. The Philistines with the help of Delilah was able to capture Samson; blind him, and make him push a grinding machine.

Samson in his conflict cried and prayed to God, and God enabled him to kill more Philistines in his death than in his life. God used Samson's bad deed by turning those bad deeds into good deeds to benefit his people." Judges 15:9 16:21 16:22-31 Holy Bible

As Samson, the feeling I am feeling is because I have been made naked. The feeling I am having is because I am depleted. The feeling I am having is because my father sinned, as his father sinned causing me to be made naked.

I was made naked at an early age. I was made naked at an early age by my father who was made naked by his father Adam. My father was made naked by his father Adam in the

Garden of Eden. My father was made naked by his father Adam in the garden because of disobediences.

My father, like Samson was warned by their Father (God) to deny the forbidden (unattainable), and if they had been obedient and listen to their Father, we all would have avoided the pitfalls that occurs when we travel down life dangerous road. God because of His Wisdom, Knowledge and Understanding always warns us of life's danger. He speaks to us more clearly now then ever before. God is with us, He looks after us; and we are His people.

And God said," let us make man in our image, after our likeness, and let them have dominion over the fish of the sea and over the fowls in the air; over the cattle and over all the earth, and over the creeping things that creeps upon the earth. So God created man in His image, in the image of God created he, male and female He created. And God blessed them and said unto them, be fruitful and multiply; and replenish the earth; subdue it and have dominion over the fish of the sea; over the fowl of the air, over every thing that moves over the earth. And the Lord took man and placed him in the Garden of Eden to dress it and to keep it. And He commanded the man saying," of every tree in the garden, thou may eat freely, but of the tree of knowledge, and good and evil, thou shall not eat there of, for in the day that thou eat there of, thou shall surely die. And then God said," it is not good that man be alone. I will make him a help mate. Then the Lord God caused a great (deep) sleep to fall upon Adam and took one of his ribs. He then closed up his flesh. And the rib that the Lord had taken from man, he made a woman and brought her unto the man, and Adam said; this is now bone of my bone and flesh of my flesh. She shall be called woman because she was taken from man. Therefore shall a man leaves his father and mother and cleave unto his wife and they shall be one flesh.

And they the man and the woman were naked and they were not ashamed. Genesis 2-13-25   Holy Bible

For a time the man and the woman were naked (undressed-unashamed-unafraid). For a time they felt no shame in their home. For a time they were as honeymooners in their home. For a time they not only talked the talk, they walked the walk, worshiped and obeyed God's commandments. They did everything that was required of them by their Father (God). They were pleased with God and God was pleased with them.

God had also placed in the garden animals, mammals, reptiles, and those that creep and crawl. Among those that creep and crawl was the most cunning of them all. This cunning serpent asked the woman (Eve) whom he knew he could coerce into doing anything," has God said to you that you shall not eat of every tree in the garden. And the woman said unto the serpent," we may eat of every fruit tree, but the fruit tree which is in the middle of the garden; God has said , we shall not eat of it, neither shall we touch it lest we die. And the Serpent said unto the woman, you shall not surely die, for your Father God does know that in the day that you eat there of the tree, then your eyes shall be opened and you shall be as the gods, knowing good and evil. And because the woman saw that the tree was good for food, and that it was pleasant and desirable to the eyes; she took of it and gave some unto her husband who desired her. And because Adam wanted to please her, he did eat also.   Genesis 3: 1-24

And they heard the voice of their Father walking and talking in the cool of the day. And Adam and his wife hid among the fig trees where they had sewed fig leaves to make Aprons." Genesis 3: 1-24

What they had done in the dark did come out in the light. Secrets and hidden things are found even when hidden in the dark. There is nothing under the sun that can be hidden from

God. If something has to be hidden from God, then it is not worth having. They the hidden things will only make us naked and ashamed.

And the Lord called Adam and said,' where art thou? And Adam said; I heard your voices in the garden, and because I was afraid (naked- ashamed) I hid from you. And the Lord asked Adam," who told you that you were naked. Hast thou eaten of the tree where of I commanded that thou not eat? And the man not taking responsibility for his actions said," the woman who thou gave me to be with, she gave me of the tree, and it looked so pleasant (delicious) so I did eat of it." Genesis 3:1-24

Adam was the first (1ST) person not to take responsibility for his action.

"And the Lord said unto the woman. Woman, what is this that thou hast done? Why did you make your husband stumble? And the woman not taking responsibility for her action said," The Serpent beguiled (deceived) me, and I did eat." Genesis 3:1-24

Eve was the second (2nd) person not to take responsibility for her action.

And the Lord said unto the Serpent," because thou has done this thing, thou art cursed above every beast of the field. Upon thy belly thou shall go; and dust shall thou eat all the days of your life; and I will put enmity between thee and the woman and between thy seed and her seed; it shall bruise thy head and thou shall bruise his heel. Genesis 3:1-24

The Serpent was the first to be cursed. He took full responsibility for his actions. He left the garden smiling because he had taken Adams and Eve's power (control). He left the garden smiling and making preparations (plans) to kill all of God's children.

"Unto the woman God said'" I will greatly multiply thy sorrow and thy conception. In sorrow shall thou bring forth children and thy husband shall rule over you." Genesis 3:16 Was Eve's punishment harsher then Adam's ?

Eve was the second (2nd) person to be cursed.

Unto Adam whose punishment wasn't as harsh as Eve, God said," because thou has harkened unto the voice of thy wife and hast eaten of the tree of which I commanded thee, saying thou shall not eat of it. Curse is the ground for thy sake. In sorrow shall thou eat of it all the days of thy life. Thorns and thistles shall it bring forth to thee and thou shall eat of the herbs of the fields. In the sweat of thy face shall thou eat bread until thou return unto the ground, for out of it was thou taken; for dust thou art, and unto dust shall thou return." Genesis 3:17-19

Adam was the third (3rd) person to be cursed.

Adam called his wife Eve because she was the mother of all living. Unto Adam and his wife did the Lord make coats of skin to clothes them, and the Lord said; the man became as one of us to know good and evil and now lest he put forth his hand and take also of the tree of life, eat it and live forever. Therefore the Lord sent Adam and Eve from the Garden of Eden (their home) to tilt the ground from whence he was taken. He drove out the man and He placed at the East of the garden of Eden a Cherubim, and a flaming sword which turned every which way to keep the way of the tree of life.

We hold the keys to our lives given to us by God. We are the master or our destiny through Christ. With God's help, we can with those keys, open doors others can not open; close doors others cannot close. He (God) alone can thereby make provision for us to be set free. All God requires of us is that we Love Him, Fear Him, Remember His commandments, Remember His creeds, principals, laws, and obey Him, and He will protect us, (safe guard us)and keep us from being ashamed of our nakedness.

Because Eve made Adam become a conspirator of her sin we then became co- conspirator of their sins.

"Jehovah Witness asked the question," Does the Bible discriminate against women? They says," that the Terrullian a thirty century Theologian once described "Women "as the devil's gate way. Others has used the Bible to portray women as less important then men. As a result, they feel that the Bible discriminates against women.

Elizabeth Cady Staton, a nineteenth Century pioneer for the rights of women in the United States felt that the Bible and the Church have been the greatest stumbling block in the way of women's emancipation; of the first five books of the Bible. Staton once said," I know of no other book that so fully teach the Subjection and Degradation of women. While some today might hold such extreme viewpoint, many still says that some parts of the Bible supports discrimination against women. Is such a conclusion justified? How women are viewed in the Hebrew Scripture," your craving will be for your husband, and he will dominate you." Genesis 3:16- Critics point to this as judgmental of Eve by God as a divine approval of women's subjection by men. However rather than a   declaration of God's purpose, this is a statement of the consequences of sin and rejection of God's sovereignty. Abuse of women is the direct results of man's kind fallen nature, and not God's will. Women in many cultures have indeed been dominated by their husbands often in very harsh ways. But this was God's purpose. Both Adam and Eve were made in God's image; moreover they received the same mandate from God to become fruitful, fill the earth, and to subdue it; they were to work together as a team. Clearly, at that point neither was dominating the other. Genesis 1:31 says," that God saw everything he had done and it was good. In some cases the Bible accounts do not indicate Gods view on the matter. They may just be historical narrative. The account of Lot's offering his daughters to the Sodomites is related without moral commentary or judgment by God. Genesis 19: 6-8 "the fact is that God hates all forms of Exploitation and Abuse. Exodus 22:22, Deut. 27:19: Isaiah 10:1-2 "The Mosaic Law condemned rape and prostitution." Leviticus 19:29, Deut. 22:22-29, Rather than discriminate against women, the law elevated and protected them from the rampant exploitation common in surrounding nations. A capable Jewish wife was a highly respected and highly esteemed individual." Proverb 3:10-30 The Israelites failure to follow God's laws of showing respect for women was their fault, not God's will. Ultimately God judged and punished the nation as a whole for their flagrant disobedience. Any society can function well only when there is order. This requires the administration of authority. The Alternative is chaos." God is a God of peace. Cor.14:33 "The Apostle Paul describes the family headship arrangement, the head of every man is Christ; in turn the head of woman is man; in turn the head of Christ is God. 1 Cor. 11:3 "Every individual except God submits to a higher authority. Does the fact that men Scripturally have been assigned to take the lead in the congregation mean that women are being discriminated against. To prosper both family and the congregation needs women and men to play their roles with love and respect. Eph. 5:21-25-28,33

Jesus consistently treated women with respect. He refused to follow the discriminatory traditions and regulation taught by the Pharisees. He talked to non- Jewish women. Matthew 15: 22-28- John 4: 7-9 – He taught women -Luke 10:10-12 – He protected women from being abandoned." Mark 10: 10-12; perhaps the most revolutionary step for His time was that

Christ accepted women into His inner circle of friends." Luke 8: 1-3 "As the perfect embodiment of all of God's qualities, Jesus showed that individuals of both sexes have equal value in God's eyes. In fact among the early Christians, both men and women received the gift of the Holy Spirit. Act 2: 14, 17-18; "For those anointed who have the prospect of serving as King and Priests with Christ there will be no distinction of gender at all once they are resurrected to the heavenly life. The Author of the Bible Jehovah does not discriminate against women." Jehovah Witness

Through Adam, sin suffering, discrimination, prison, darkness, and death came into the world. Through Jesus, life resurrection, redemption, justice, salvation, and grace came into the world.

There is a prison that we lock ourselves into and don't have the ability (key) to get ourselves out of ; and there is another prison that man locks us into which isn't easy to exit (as Joseph), because they alone holds that key.

"Joseph the son of Jacob found himself locked into prison because of jealousy created by his Father. Jacob loved all of his sons, but favored Joseph because of his love for Rachel. Joseph Brother's (siblings) sold him to a company of men (Israelites) going from Gilead to Egypt for twenty pieces of silver. He later was sold to Portimar and became the ruler of Portimar's house. He resisted the advances of Portimars wife who tried to make him naked, and was cast into prison. Joseph later comforts his brothers and father and promised them that the Lord would bring them out of Egypt (slavery)." Genesis 37:40 and 50

It is never easy to exit the prison of the flesh. It is never easy to exit the prison of the flesh until they decide that we have been incarcerated long enough as Joseph found out once he lost his freedom. Before Adam was tempted (tested), he held the key (control) to his life which gave him the option (power over the devil) as to whether he would eat from the tree or not. When my father was tempted, he also had the power of not eating from the tree. The Bible says," that man does not live by bread alone, but by every word that comes from the mouth of God. The word of God will be the key to our power; the key to our control.

God had programmed Adam to resist the devil. God had also programmed my dad to resist the devil and be obedient, but because they let the devil dictate who they were, I am also programmed now to sin. When Adam sinned in the garden, the sin he committed was passed on to my father. When my father sinned outside of the garden, the sin he committed was passed on to me. When I sinned outside of the garden, the sins I committed was passed on to my children (grandchildren). The cycle is now being passed on to the next generation. If Adam and my father had been obedient to their Father (God), we all would have been safe and secure in our Father arm, but because they lacked the wisdom, knowledge and understanding needed to adhere to the policies of God. We are all now, without shelter from the storm, "for resplendent and unfading wisdom she is readily perceived by those who love her. She hurries to make herself known in anticipation of their desire. For taking thought of wisdom is the protection of prudence and whoever for her own sake keep virtue, shall quickly be safe from care. Because she makes her own rounds, seeking those worthy of her and graciously appears to them in the ways that meet them in solitude." Wisdom 8:12-16

After the garden, Adam and Eve had no choice but to go on living. The difference was that they had a different way of life, a different life style outside the garden then inside the garden.

Outside the garden, they lived a life of pain, suffering, and heartaches rather than a life that their Father had vision for them. God had vision a life of peace, joy, happiness and growth.

After the garden, Adam and Eve had children (Cain and Abel). Abel had a love for his family (God), while Cain had no regard for his family (God)." For Fidelity of Yahweh implies many particular virtues; and among them Sirah gives precedents of duty toward the parents, He promises atonement for sin to those who honor their parents." Sir 3:2-7, 12-14

"God set a father over His children; a mother authority He confirms over His sons; whoever honors his father atones for his sins and preserve himself. When we pray we are heard; we store up riches for those who honor our mother. Whoever obeys his father will live a long life; He obeys his father, he who brings comfort to the mother. My son, take care of the father when he is old; grieve him not all the days of his life as long as he lives. Even if his mind fails him, ye should be considerate of him. Ye shall revive him not all the days of his life. Kindness and love to the father will not be forgotten, firmly planted against the debt of your sins, a house raised to you in justice." Sirach 3:27

Cain didn't know that," a wise son make a glad father, but a foolish son is heaviness to his mother, nor did he hear the instruction of his father, and forsake not the instruction of his mother." Proverb 1-10

Cain and Abel weren't born in the original garden. And even though they weren't born in the original garden they still had a chance to turn a bad situation into a good situation. All they had to remember was that God is the master of our destination and only He can sustain us no matter what garden we were born in, for He guards the course of the just and protects the way of His faithful." Proverb 2:18

Because of the sins committed in the garden, my father wasn't allowed in the origin garden either, and because he didn't try to make the best of a bad situation, my eyes were then opened and I was made naked and ashamed, all because of the forbidden (unattainable).

Jehovah Witness says," that although Paradise was lost Jehovah gives hope. The very prophesy of the Bible speaks of a seed who will undo the effect of sin and bruise Satan in the head. Genesis 3:15

Due to the bitterness of the Serpent, he decided that he would make all God's children pay for what God had done to him. He had been kicked out of Heaven and kicked out of the garden. He then decided to make Adam and Eve pay through their children. Satan tormented Cain, made him jealous and made him disobey his father Adam and his Father God. This is how sibling rivalry first came into the world with our children. Cain didn't hear the words of our Father which said," my son, if sin (Satan) entice you, consent not; walk not thou in the way with him; refrain thy foot from his path, for his feet run to evil, and make haste to shed blood." Proverb1:10-16

How was Cain to know that to kill was not of God, his parents had already killed once they had sinned in the garden by being disobedient. They thereby made it easy for all of us to sin. Cain listened to Satan and killed his younger brother Abel. He killed Abel because he was jealous and wasn't chosen by God.

Cain was the first one to commit murder upon another human being, he didn't take full responsibility for his action, and yet he asked God to have mercy on him. Was it fair of God to choose the younger brother as His favorite making Cain jealous?

God was the first (1st) parent to set the guidelines (examples) for the children (Adam-Eve), which was good. Adam and Eve were the second (2nd) parents to set the guidelines for the children, which wasn't good. And due to the negative example that they (Adam-Eve) set, I didn't have a good foundation to go by either.

Sin accosted me at an early age. I had sin tattooed on me when I entered into the world and sin has continued to follow me now thanks to my ancient fathers. I then received (inherited) sin through my father.

My dad and my mom met through their job at a shrimp factory. They connected with each other, married, and had children as God had ordained them. "After the doings of the land of Egypt, they did not do the things of the land of Canaan, neither did they walk in their ordinances; they did God's judgment and kept God ordinance, to walk there in because of the Lord their God. They therefore kept His statues and His judgment which if we do, we shall live. The Lord is the Lord and none shall approach to any that is near to Him to uncover their nakedness; God is the Lord. The nakedness of the mother shall thou not uncover. The daughter of thy father or the daughter of thy mother, whether she is born at home or born abroad, even her nakedness, they shall not uncover." Leviticus 18: 1-18

We as a society must be mindful (less tolerant) of the things that we (others) do. Fr. Paul McQuillen- St. Joseph the Worker Catholic Church

William Rasberry says," a friend of his was saying how remarkable it is that many of us seem to have found the right mates, not paragons, but people who possess the qualities that are important to us and make our lives more complete. He says that he suggested this possibility that maybe it isn't their wonderful qualities that make us see those we've chosen to marry, perhaps it the marriage that makes us see those qualities.

He thought that it was fresh until a reason conversation with David Blankenhorn.

Blankenhorn called Rasberry's attention to a letter Theologian Dietrich Bonhoeffer had written in a Nazi prison cell to a young bride and groom in 1943." Your love is your own private possession Bonhoeffer told the young couple, it is a status; an office. It is not your love that sustains the marriage, but for now, the marriage that sustains your love.

Rasberry says," if this seems subject for an op-ed column, the truth is that almost everything he touches these days impels him to consider the troubled institution of marriage. He thinks of this when he sees many Duke University Students settling for uncommitted relationship; living together or merely "hook -up," He say's he thinks of this when he see young children struggling academically because their mother are unable to give them economic, emotional, directional support they need; He thinks of this when he sees young boys running amok, and young men over populating our prisons in large part because they haven't had the loving discipline that father's can provide. And he thinks of this when he see young and not so young men who can't seem to make sense of their role in modern life. As often happens Rasberry say's when he thinks of these things he calls Blankenhorn (President of the institute for American values and a leader of what has been dubbed the Marriage movement)

When Rasberry calls Blankenhorn in New York Blankenhorn says," that he Rasberry shouldn't be surprised at the sense of rootlessness and directionlessness especially among young males, after all, we've been saying for generations that father's aren't really necessary. What is so shocking is that some are starting to believe." William Rasberry Times Picayune

I was the oldest of two daughters; the oldest of many cousins, born to a mother and father who was married. Three months after I was born, my mom became pregnant again and my dad because of the depression decided that he would leave his job at the shrimp factor in New Orleans and go to Detroit to seek employment. When my dad left Louisiana, It was decided that he would go to Detroit; find employment, then relocate my mom; myself and the new baby once she was born. My dad was successful in Detroit, he did find a job (Ford Motor Company); and then something went amok. Something went amok and my dad forgot to relocate his ready made family that God had given him.

My father forgot about us, married someone else; and had four (4) others children. He chose another woman, another marriage, another family, was this fair (obedient of him)? My mother was supposed to be bone of his bone, flesh of his flesh. She was called woman because she had been taken from man." Genesis 3:7

My father left his father and his mother to cleave to a wife (my mother), and they should have been as one flesh. God didn't intend for him to have two (2) flesh. Genesis 3:7

My parent should not have been naked and ashamed, but because my father wanted the unattainable like Samson and like Adams; but because my father was tempted (tested), and ate of the forbidden his eyes was made open and he was made ashamed (naked). God had gone before him to keep him on the right path. God said," I have made thee in thy way of Wisdom, Knowledge and Understanding; I have led thee in the right path so that when thou goes, then thou steps shall not straitened; and when thou run thou shall not stumble. Proverb 4: 1-19

My father when he stumble he then defined who I was supposed to become. I then became the naked (ashamed and abandon) child who was made to sin. I then was not worthy to be compared with the glory to be reveled to me; for I was made subject to vanity, not willingly, but by reason of him who hast subjected it; and because I shall not be delivered from bondage during this life time, I didn't wait for the redemption of my body. I didn't wait to be redeemed. Roman 8:18-22

A Redeemer (Redemption) is something that is beyond my comprehension. I only saw my mother and yearn for my father, because my father was no where's to be found. If it takes a tribe to raise a village, where has my tribe gone? My father has gone astray with no concept as to what he had done. He took pleasure for a little while for himself, and ignored the damage he caused when he made the decision to flee.

Because of my father's action, his Father (God) will have to deem it necessary to send a repairman (Jesus) to clean up his mess, because we are all now creatures of the dark with no one to rescue us.

Adam and my father were made in the image of God, so what went wrong (amok) with their makeup.   Genesis 1:27

"Jehovah say's, being in the image of God, human's have the capacity to reflect God's attributes. Surely we want to cultivate such qualities as Love, Mercy, Goodness, Kindness, and Patience, reflecting the One who made us."   Genesis 1:26   Marriage is God's arrangement. The Marriage bond is permanent and sacred, with the husband serving as head of the house."   Genesis 2:22-24   Happiness is dependent on our recognizing Jehovah's sovereignty in our life. Jehovah's words always come true."   Genesis 3:18-19, 5:5, 6-7-23

My father had a ready made family, a true wife, but for whatever reason, the family that he had already just wasn't good enough for him. For when God joined my dad and my mom together, he told them, not to let anyone tare them asunder. Because when one finds a worthy wife, her value is far beyond pearls. Her husband entrusting his heart to her has an unfailing prize. She brings him good and not evil all the days of her life. She obtains wool and flax and works with loving hands. She puts her hands to the distaff and her fingers to the spindle. Sunday Missal

At birth because of our parents (mother and father), we should have been born with the faith to trust someone. We should have been born with the faith to truth our mother and father; we should have been born with the faith to trust God. In life faith is words in deed only. It must be carried out in action. Words alone will not cover the naked, nor will it give food to the hungry; for what good is it to say that we have faith if our actions do not prove (show) it.

Because of my father, I don't have the faith to trust anyone. God believed (trusted) in Adam, and he betrayed Him. My mom trusted (believe) in my dad, and he betrayed her; those who place their trust (faith) in man are bound to fail. Those who place their trust in God shall inherit the earth.

Was there a flaw in my father that my mother didn't see? Was there a flaw in him that made him go against God will? Was there a flaw in him that made him decide that he wasn't going to return to Louisiana? Was there a flaw in him that made him stay in Detroit, marry another; and kept that secret from his first (1st) wife and his second (2nd) wife? So many questions, so many lies; he had the gift of choice (as Adam), but he did not choose God's will, he chose to go the way of the flesh. He chose to sin instead.

"Jane Pic wrote," that she recently had read a parable and thought she would share it. It tells the story of an elderly Chinese woman who carried two large pots of water on the end of a pole she held across her neck. One pot had a crack in it, but the other was perfect. As she trudged backward and forward daily from the well where she dipped the pots in the water to carry back to the house, she noticed that when she arrived home the cracked pot had only half the amount of the water in it than when she began to walk, but the other pot was still full. This went on for a couple of years. The pot with the crack was ashamed of its imperfection and miserable that it did only half of what it was made to do. Finally it spoke to the old woman and said, I am ashamed of myself because this crack on my side caused water to leak out all the way back to the house. The old woman smiled and said," Did you not noticed that there are flowers on your side of the path but not on the other size of the path? She went on to explain that because of its flaws she planted seeds on the side of the path, and everyday as they walked home, the seeds were watered and nourished and that because of the pot, she could pick beautiful flowers to decorate her table. Without you being just the way you are there would not be this beauty to grace my house. The parable continues; each of us has our own unique flaw. But it's the cracks and flaws we each have that make our lives together so very interesting and rewarding. You just have to take each for what they are and for the good in them." Jane Pic- Times Picayune

Adam was made in God's likeness (flawless), and became flawed because of sin. He was made in God's image and because he sinned, there came a flaw in my father and that flaw was passed on to me.

"Bishop Noel Jones say's that," sin is transferred to us through our parents. It sin is like a wire (money) transfer that is transferred from one account to another. He also says that we need to stop living in sin and live in righteousness, because righteousness is where the power lies." Bishop Noel Jones

After my father exit from our lives, life continued to move on as it did when Adam and Eve exit the garden. My mom stilled had two (2) babies to feed, support and care for. She still had to make sure that all of our needs were met. She decided after my sister was born to return to the cold, damp, shrimp factory to ensure that the bills were paid and our needs were met.

After a period of time my mom met someone else. There was a depression (recession), and there was only so much that he could do for her ready made family.

My mom became pregnant again and then not only did she have three (3) mouths to feed, she then had four (4) mouths to feed plus some of her sibling as well.

After my brother was born, my mom returned to the cold, damp, dreary shrimp factory where my grandmother had contacted Tuberculosis and died.. My mom returned to the shrimp factory where she contacted tuberculosis also.

My mom died on April 1, 1953. My mom died jut shy of me reaching six years old. My mom died before she had reached the age of thirty years old. I didn't comprehend until much later the magnitude of the pain and suffering she must have endured. I didn't think about how she must have felt as the lepers in the Bible who were ill with taboo (terrible illnesses). I now feel the isolation (loneliness) she must have felt because of her illness. She was as the Israelites whom the Lord spoke of to Moses (Aaron). He said," when any man hath a running issue out of his flesh, because of his issue he is unclean and this shall be his uncleanness in his issue; whether his flesh run with his issue, or his flesh be stopped from his issue, it is uncleanness. If you touch the bed he lies on; if you sit on the things he hath set on that has the issue, if you touch the flesh; If he spit on you, you shall wash your clothes, and bath in the water and be unclean until the even."   Leviticus 15:1-3

I now realize that I have a prolong anger for my father. I now realize that I have a prolong anger against my father because he wasn't there for my mom when she needed him the most. I now realize that I didn't need a father after all.

I remember my mom. I remember my mom as if it was yesterday. I remember living on Sere Street, and my mom taking me to our neighbor's (Ms. Elvee) house to get my ear's pierced for the very first time.

I remember living on Orleans Street in our baby bed my sister fighting me and my mom having to separate us. I remember my mom pushing me in a rocking chair backward and forward, and making sure that I didn't fall out of it. I remember my mom taking me to School to place me in the Kindergarten program at the age of three (3) years old. I remember the fat little bully who took my emerald necklace from around my neck and how I cried because my mom had given it to me. I remember, oh how I remember. I remember how I used to stick under my mother. I remember how I used to stick under my mom like glue before she died. I remember how I didn't want her to go anywhere's without me.

My grandmother preceded my mother in death by a couple of years or so. She had worked in the shrimp factory as my mom trying to make a living also. The only memory I have of my grandmother is my mom and her siblings taking care of their mom until she died from tuberculosis.

My grandfather preceded my grandmother in death by a couple of years or so. I am told that I was the oldest baby when he died. My grandfather who died prior to my grandmother committed Suicide. When I asked my aunts and uncles why he had done such a thing, I am told that it was probably because he was sick and tired of his suffering and pain.

I remember the day that my mom died. I remember how I woke up screaming and howling; and my aunt coming in my room to asked me what was wrong with me; and because I was afraid of her I didn't answer her. She then told me to get up and get ready for School.

On the day that my mom died, a neighbor boy by the name of Jimmy came up to me after school and told me that my mom had died and because it was April's Fool Day, I didn't want to believe that my mother was dead. I slowly walked home; I slowly reached the block that I lived on, and when I reached the block; I saw a black hearse sitting in front of the door.

I was in denial, I was in a trance; I went in a trance because I didn't want to believe that my friend, my protector; my companion; my savior was gone. I didn't want to believe that the only person I had ever trusted; the only person I had ever believed in had died and left me all alone.

I didn't know or realize at that time it would be a long time before I would be safe, secure and unafraid. I didn't know that God would have to send a redeemer (His only Son) to save me and make me safe and secure. I didn't realize at that time that God is indeed my Savior, I should not be afraid. My strength and courage is the Lord, and He has been my Savior, with joy I shall draw water at the fountain of Salvation. I didn't give thanks to the Lord; I didn't acclaim His Holy name among the nations or make known his deeds or proclaim how exalted His Holy name is. I didn't sing praise to the Lord for His glorious achievement, or let any of this be known through out all the earth, nor shout with exultation (O city o Zion) for great in our midst is really the Holy One."

On the day of the Funeral, my dad was no where's to be found. Many letters had been sent to my people in Eudora (Arkansas). Many letters were sent to Eudora and no one took the time to acknowledge them. No one would even give information as to where he really was. I didn't ask God why my dad had left me. I didn't ask God Why my mom had left me and never came back. I just went to my prison cell for my first (1st) imprisonment. I just went to my cave (coffin), never to return emotionally for a very long time. I just joined my mom in her coffin, never to return until my Father (God) sent Jesus, His Only Son (Advocate-Redeemer) to rescue me.

At the cemetery everyone took their places at the grave site. Everyone went where they needed to go to put my mom in her grave. There was a pile of dirt already waiting. There was a pile of dirt waiting to be thrown over her once she was placed in the ground. I couldn't go near the burial site. I couldn't go near the burial site because I didn't want to believe that she was dead.

I didn't know how long it would be before I feel any emotion. I didn't know how long it would be before I feel any grief. I just knew that it would be the last time I would see my mother again. I just knew that I was headed for jail.

After my mom died, my mom's siblings went back into their routine (survival). Some of them went back to work; some of them went off to school and others stayed home to care for the younger children in the house. Once my mom died many things changed. Many things changed and the changes weren't for the better.

Due to my dad's desertion; due to my mother's death, my siblings and myself went into prison (Egypt as Joseph). We were placed in prison because there were those who didn't fear the Lord," For the fear of the Lord is clear, enduring forever. The law of the Lord is perfect (refreshing)," and those who doesn't fear the Lord just don't grow.

For my sibling and my self to grow and become who God had intended for us to become, our foundation needed to be firm (solid). If the foundation is solid, the building will be solid; if the foundation is decompose; the building will decompose. A building can not be built with unreliable material and then expected to endure. The foundation (soil) I was placed in was not strong (solid) from the beginning, so I was not made strong. There were many problems prior to my grandfather (grandmother) dying. There were many problems after my father left; there were many problems after my mother died, and there are just as many problems now. The soil I was place in, even though it looked good on the outside had too much sand and not enough rocks (like the levee) to enable me to stand on solid ground. The soil (foundation) I was placed in was not solid enough for me to endure," for everyone who listen to the words of the Lord (God), fears Him and acts on His words will be as the wise man who built his house on solid rocks. The rain will fall, the flood waters will come, and the wind will blow and buffed the house. But the house will not collapse because it has been placed solidly on rocks. And everyone who listen to the words of God and does not act on them will be as the fool who built his house on sand. The rain felled, the flood water rolled, the wind blew and buffed the house, causing the house to collapse and be completely destroyed.

Sibling rivalry was first started with Cain and Abe. (Genesis 4:4-26); it was in effect with Joseph and his brothers (Genesis 37:1-6; it was in effect with my aunts and uncles (my sister and me), and it is still in effect so many years later. The enemy (devil) lurks on every side anxious and ready to take vengeance on us.

"Jeffery Kluger say's," that for a long time researchers have tried to nail down just what shapes us, or what at least shapes us the most. And over the years, they've had a lot of eureka moments. First it was our parents, particularly our mother; then it was our genes; next it was our peers who showed up last but hold sway. And all these ideas went platinum. The fact is once investigation had strip all the data from the theories they still came away with as many questions as answers. Somewhere there was a sort of temperamental dark matter exerting on invisible gravitational pull of its own. More and more Scientist are concluding that this unexplained force is our siblings. From the time they are born, our brothers and sisters are our collaborators and conspirators; our role models and cautionary tales. They are our scolds, protectors, goads, tormentors, playmates, counselors, source of envy, object of pride. They teach us how to conduct friendships and when to walk away from them. Sisters teach brothers about the mysteries of girls and brothers teach sisters about the puzzles of boys. Our spouses arrive comparatively late in our lives, our parents eventually leaves us. Our siblings may be the only people we'll ever know who truly qualifies as partners for life. Siblings says family Sociologist Katherine Conger of the University of California," sibling are with us for the whole Journey." Jeffery Kluger

Children learn what they see, hear and feel from their parents. As the parent teaches the children how to walk, talk, crawl, eat, etc, so shall they teach them how to get alone with others. If the parent relationship is out of control then the children relationship with others will be out of control also. There will be no peace.

"Bishop T.D. Jakes says," that the Lord gives us all the gift of Peace; and when that peace is gone, it is usually because there is a bump (pot hole) in the road. There is usually something interfering with their gift of peace." Bishop TD Jakes.

There was a bump in the road on Sere Street. In the house on Sere Street, there was a division; there was a breakup; there was no peace. The division started taring (separating) the family apart. "They forgot about God's mercy; they forgot about God's grace; they forgot God's kindness and forgot about His gentleness. They let the enemies triumph over their yesterday, and gave them access to their today and tomorrow." Psalm 25:6

They forgot in their mourning and weeping to seek God; they forgot in their despair that weeping endures for a night, but joy cometh in the morning. They were all to busy trying to take control and eventually lost control. They didn't humble themselves and seek God, nor did they ask Him not to hide from them. They neither knew that when their mother and father had died that the Lord would be the one to take them up. Psalm 27:10 Sunday Missal

Life was only tolerable for the siblings and orphans on Sere Street. Life was only tolerable and the burden of trying to feed everyone during a depression was too great. Life then became unbearable. I didn't ask God Why? I asked how long was these suffering and pain going to end.

My aunt kept trying to get in touch with my dad, using the information he had left behind in case of an emergency. But the information didn't help much because my dad didn't want to be found. The information that was given to my mom was information (phone –address) on my paternal side of the family. They my grandparents in Eudora knew where my dad was, they just wasn't sharing that information with my maternal side of the family. From time to time one of my father's brothers had been in touch with my mom before her death. After she died there was no more contact (communication).

Tension continued to mount in the little house on Sere Street. Tension existed because there were too many living in the small cramped house; too many mouths to feed; too many bills to pay; to many trying to take control and not enough money to cover the whole tribe (village); then to make matters worse; then to add less fuel to the fire that was already burning out of control, my aunt (our) life changed and not for the better.

My aunt met a man and felled in love. The man my aunt met was a taxi cab driver; a taxi cab driver who later became a minister (monster). My aunt met a monster who would make all our lives worst than what it was." For the Lords warns His people not to oppress the foreign, nor to harm the widows and the orphans, that consideration for the poor and needy should be their prime concern." My aunt's new fellow didn't hear the words of the Lord because of Spiritual weakness.

Tension got worse in the poor cramped house, fuel continue to burn and to add fuel to the fire, the minister (monster) eventually moved into the poor, cramped, crowded, pack filled house, changing the compose. It also changed the tone and mood, making life unbearable for all who lived there.

Niger John as he was called started taking over and making life miserable. Life was so unbearable that slowly my uncles and aunts started moving out one by one. They did just what he wanted them to do; he wanted them all to move out so that he could go on with his next plan. My brother who was born later than my sister and me was moved to Opelousas by Rev's mother house and life became a little better for him.

Life was just getting started for the two sisters on Sere Street. My sister and I had to endure many hardships, sufferings, hurts and pains .We suffered more because we didn't have anyone to rescue us; we were the orphans that no one looked out for. My cousins faired out better; they faired out because their mothers were in and out of the house and made a point of checking on them.

My sister had life harder than I did. She had life harder because she fought the abuses. She would run to the neighbors house naked, and my aunt (uncle) would tell the police when they were called by the neighbors that the reason for her nakedness was because she had done something wrong and when they had tried to discipline her for her actions, she would run to the neighbors house for protection. Our neighbors helped us out a lot, but there was only so much help they could give us.

We went to Church often. We went to Church from Sunday to Saturday, and since we were the pillow of society, we were expected to be in Church every time the doors were open.

Life was horrible in the house; so much so that two (2) of the younger brothers went off into the military to get out of the house. The youngest of the three brothers eventually went into the military also. They went into the Military to escape from the house of secrets. They went into the Military to escape the house of the monster.

Just about all the unwanted family members are out of the house on Sere Street now. Niger John has accomplished what he set out to do. The castle is his for the taking. He is now lord of the manor; he can now do what he set out to do. He can now molest (undress) the two orphan sister's with out any interference (confrontation) from the natives.

Rev started molesting my sister and me at an early age. He could do so freely because he had rid the playing field of all its adversaries. He could do so freely because he had made sure that the neighbors wouldn't interfere anymore.

My sister had life harder. She had life harder because she fought the abuses while I gave into the abuses. The reason my situation was easier was because I didn't rebel (act out-act aggressive). The reason my situation was easier was because I gave in and didn't run to the neighbor house for cover. I realize early in the ball game that it was easier for me if I gave in to the abuses, then if I fought the abuses. I decided to try my mother's approach of making lemonade with the lemon's that was given to her. I learned to adjust to the situation. I learned to make lemonade with the situation while dealing with the abuses (nakedness).

My dad leaving and my mom dying made for a perilous (bad) situation. My sister and I were left in prison naked trying to make since of a bad situation. I still didn't ask God why did this (curse) happen? I only asked Him, how long do I have to make lemonade?

Life in prison didn't get any better. On many occasions on my way to school, I had to stand by one of the apartment buildings in the project and try to compose myself before going to school. My nerves would be shot and my stomach would be killing me. Going home after school was harder because I never knew when Rev would send my aunt on one of her many errands or when he would at night creep into my room. On many occasions when the others were asleep, he would take me in the kitchen and do what he wanted to me. I was afraid to cry out to anyone just as at my mom funeral. I was afraid to cry out because there was no one to rescue me (like my sister); there was no one to hear me, there was no one to help us in our time of need.

Because the house had so many secrets, there were only a little bit of activities for my sister and me. The only outside activities was Church and at School. If there was something going on after School and we were required to participate, my aunt would accompany us so that we wouldn't spill any of the family jewels (secrets).

And then at the age of sixteen (12) grade after being abuse for approximately nine (9) years, I had had enough. I had had enough of the abuses (physical-mental-verbal-sexual). I had had enough of the undressing (nakedness), and finally I got the nerves to tell my aunt what Niger John had been doing to me.

My aunt knew that Rev was evil; my aunt knew that Rev wasn't a man of God; my aunt knew that Rev wasn't who he pretended to be on the outside. On the outside he was suppose to be a minister, but on the inside he lacked the Spiritual Healing (peace) that only God (Jesus) can give. My aunt knew that Rev was molesting my sister and me and was having sex with many females in the Sanctuary of the Church. My aunt instead of taking her frustration (pain-suffering) out on him took her hurt and pain out on my sister and me. She was in denial; she was in love, she was hurting on the inside and acting out on the outside. She was as the brook that dried up from lack of water. She had dried up from lack of attention. She had dried up because of lack of faith in God." She didn't know that Jesus gives us strength to preserve. God calls His followers into the Friendship of Christ." Sunday Missal

My aunt was the brook that dried up because the man she loved was too busy molesting little girls and having affairs in the Church with his choir members, ushers and etc, to give her the attention that she needed, and because she was feeling neglected and abused, (used)), she decided to take her frustrations and abuses out on my sister and me. I didn't ask God why? I just asked how long.

We went to Church on the same night I had told my aunt of the abuses. When we entered Church Rev (niger John) started picking on me about something I was supposed to have done. I was so tired by then of what I had been going through in the house on Sere Street (Gibson Street- St. Bernard Project) as well as in the Church, the little timid scared girl just snapped and told him in the Church that I was tired of his shi?, and I ran out of the Church and hid in the bushes.

He sent someone after me, and I was scared to death that they would find me. Due to the fact that it was dark and the Lord was on my side, they weren't able to find me. When I thought I was safe, I ran and ran to a friend from School house to see if I could get them to help me. My friend helped me catch a bus and I went to another sister of my mother 's house.

My aunt when I arrived at her house called Rev and my aunt (her sister) to let them know where I was and that I was safe. The police became involved and I was sent back into prison. I was sent back into prison because I was afraid to tell the Police what had been happening to my sister and me on Gibson Street. I was sent back because I was afraid they wouldn't believe me as they hadn't believed my sister (the neighbor's) when she had tried to tell the police what they had been doing to her.

When I returned to the house, Rev tried to intimidate me. He tried to intimidate me as if I was his possession. He tried to intimidate me, but for some reason or another, I wasn't afraid of him anymore. I stood my ground. I stood my ground because God had made me hard hearted (headed) as He had done to Pharaoh with the Israelites in Egypt (Red Sea).

The following Sunday after I was brought back to the house, my sister and I went to Sunday School (Church), and I told her to go on because I wasn't going. I told her I was leaving and she had to make up her mind what she was going to do.

I left her on her way to Church, and I took the money given to me for Sunday School and went to the same aunt's house I had gone to before; but this time was different with different results. This time I told my aunt I couldn't stay in the same house with Rev and my aunt because they were abusing us; they were assaulting (attacking- striking) my sister and me. My aunt this time called her older brother, my uncle and told him how Rev and my aunt had been abusing me and my sister and when Rev this time came to take his possession from my aunt's house, my uncle told him what he was going to do to him if he tried to remove me. Rev realizing that this battle wasn't his for the taking, this battle was the Lord's tucked his tail between his leg and fled, not looking like the head but like the tail.

I had cried and prayed for many years on the inside (inwardly), and God heard my cry and decided that I had had enough. He decided to rescue me by way of the Red Sea. God had not caused my suffering, he had not caused my pain, but he let the abuses happen to see what I would do; what I would do when my back was up against the wall.

What had happened to me and my siblings was because of the disobedience of Adam and Eve. What had happened to us was because of the disobedience of my father; what had happened to us was because of the disobedience of Rev and my aunt, eventually my sister, brother and I escaped Egypt by way of the Red Sea.

God had taken us out of Egypt (Prison-captivity). He made Pharaoh hardhearted, but our freedom was short lived. Our captivity did not last long. Our captivity was just the beginning because we next went into the captivity of our own making. We then went into captivity for forty (40) years.

When we siblings exited Egypt, God had made all the necessary accommodations for our trip, but due to the fact that we had been in prison (Egypt) for so long a period of time, we exited the Red Sea with a slave man's mentality. We weren't prepared for the freedom of the wilderness.

We crossed into the wilderness for a new life which should have been a blessing, rather than a curse; which should have been a time of renewal (rejoicing), instead we took an old mentally into a new world because we were afraid of the giants of the land.

We went into the wilderness wandering round and round for forty (40) years, trying to make sense of what had happened to us. The three of us went into the wilderness dead because of sin; dead because of nakedness, and because we hadn't received the anointing of God, we went further out of Gods protection into Satan's welcome arms; into Satan arms of protection.

Over the years, my sister and I haven't gotten any closer. We are at odds with each other all the time. She felt and still feel that I am responsible for everything that happened to her, and that I was treated better than she was.

My brother was real young when my mother died. His father was in and out of his life; until his death. When he finished High School he went into the military (Viet Nam War). He was able to escape Rev's and my aunt war, but wasn't able to escape the flesh man's war (prison), because he didn't have anyone to run interference for him with the draft board; and add to that he was shot in VietNam; some of his friends were killed in Viet Nam; he was a part of Agent Orange he still haven't emotionally been able to apply for his benefits.

I ran away at sixteen, married at seventeen; and had my first child just shy of my eighteenth birthday. Due to my leaving Egypt with so many issues, and not telling anyone (my husband) about my abuses (past), my marriage and my life fell apart. Upon my marriage falling apart because of depression (despondencies-melancholy), I took my children on my joy ride with me. All the problems of ancient time (old- of the pass) has been handed down to them. I took the old dough and the old yeast with me as the Israelites did when fleeing Egypt; ruining the new products (fruits) that God had given me.   Exodus 12:34

I learned from the past, how not to have faith and trust in anyone, and that is the inheritance that my children received from me; that is their legacy." I didn't know that the Lord keep faith forever, secure justice for the oppressed; and give food to the hungry. I didn't know that He sets prisoners free." Psalms 146:7 I also didn't know that He gives sight to the blind, lift those who are bowed down: loves the gracious and the righteous, watched over the alien and sustains the fatherless and the widows, but He frustrates the way of the wicked. The lord reins forever, Your God, O Zion, for all generation. Psalm 146:7-9

Finally I went over into the land of promise (Canaan), the land that was promised to Abraham, Isaac, Jacob and Joseph. God only required a few things: a few important things once

I entered Canaan. With all the insane (crazy things) I had been through, God was hoping that I was ready (humble-matured enough) to do His will. I should have been docile as a child (puppy). All He required of me was that I love Him, fear Him, and live according to His laws and decrees given to us by Moses (Joshua). He also asked me to rid the land of the people (idol gods) living in the land." Instead of doing what He asked me to do, I chose to do just the opposite. I chose to live amongst the enemies in the land and chose to live their life style. It wasn't that I didn't love God when I sinned, it was just that I didn't have any concept of what love was; what obedience, trust and faith was. The only thing I did know was how to get naked and undressed.

In Canaan, I did what God knew I would do; instead of what He hoped I would do. In Canaan, I went the way of the wicked instead the way of God. I lied, cheated, stole (ball point pens, newspapers, Mae Walker Rosaries Beads, too many husbands), committed adultery and even had an abortion. I lived amongst the naked (flesh)) and became just as unclean as they had become, just the opposite of God's will. He wanted me to be different from the other inhabitants. Ephesians 5: 17-20 Holy Bible

In Canaan, the inhabitants didn't have any concept of right or wrong. They had been doing what they had wanted to do so long, that they thought it was alright to disregard God's commandments and cling to human traditions. From them came Evil thoughts, thief, murder, adultery, greed malice, deceit, licentiousness, envy, blasphemy, arrogance, folly. All of these evils were coming from their heart and they defied God."

They defied God's laws not realizing that all of God's laws, decrees, and commandments are important. They felt that they could separate one sin from another sin, not realizing that a sin, is a sin, is a sin, and all are falling short of the grace of God in not believing his words." For a believing Faith comes from God. The proof of loving God comes from observing His commandments. The Spirit of Truth will testify to this," Because by grace, God will appear, saving all and training all to reject godless ways, and worldly desires and to live temperately, justly and devoutly in this age." Titus 22:11-24   Holy Bible

Instead we isolate God's commandment to fit our own needs. We look at the sins of others to minimize (play down) the sins we commit. When we suffer it is usually because of the choices that we make. We sin because we want to do what others do. We sin for the benefit of sinning as Adam, as my father; or as PFC Lynndie England who said," I had a choice to do right in the Ghraib case, but I chose to do what my friends wanted. Peer pressure was used as blame in that case. Baltimore Times (Times Picayune)- Gail Gibson

God is the mold in which we should pattern our lives. Instead we choose by choice to go against what He stands for because we are afraid of alienating ourselves and others. We use God's words for our own purpose (use) even though we know it is wrong.

I went through life doing much of the same things that the inhabitants of Canaan did because I was afraid of aliening them; afraid of loosing their respect; I didn't want them to think less of me because I had been made naked and ashamed. I didn't want them to know that I had many hidden secrets.

I was made to sin (of sin), and God knew what I would do once I was in Canaan. He (God) said," this girl will rise up and go a whoring after the gods of the strangers of the land who she has gone to be among (with) and will forsake Me, and break my covenant which I have with her; then my anger will (shall) be kindled against her and her children and I will hide my face from her and she shall be devoured; and many evils (troubles) shall fall on her so that she will say in that day," are not these evils come upon me because my God is not with me anymore." Holy Bible

Because I conform to the idol gods and other nations; and because I became just like them, God hid His face from me and delivered me up for my guilt, and it has consumed me. "Isaiah 64:7

Because I had done the crime (evil deed), God hid His face from me and left me all alone. I had never been so alone in all my life. I then was returned to the time that my father had left me; I was then returned to the time that my mother had left me (died);I then was returned to the time when I didn't have any one to rescue me. I then was returned to the time when I didn't have any one but those who had undressed me and made me naked.

When God abandon me, I then realize the dept of my sorrow (pain). I then realized that I had lost the one Father who had loved me, protected me; rescue me; safe guard me, I then realized that I had lost the One Father who had carried me through all my aches and pains. I then knew for a certainty that I was naked, alone and afraid.

Birds have a way of tending to their young (babies) long before they are born (hatched). These birds builds nest to place their eggs in, and sits on the eggs (nest) until they are hatched. The mother and the father then takes turn sitting on the nest to provide them with support, nourishment, love and protection. Once the babies (birds) are born, the parents continue to support them until they fly off on their own into the sunset and, that is how God our Father provides support, protection, and nourishment to us.

I wasn't as strong as the birds, I wasn't strong (courageous) enough to follow and observe the Laws which God commanded. I turned to the right. I turned to the left and in doing so, I didn't prosper whither I go.

When God left me, I knew something was wrong, but what I didn't know was that He had broken me. I didn't know that I had had a nervous breakdown (July 1999). I just thought I was exhausted; I just thought that I needed some rest; I just thought that I needed a break (some sleep). I wouldn't accept the fact that God had made me naked (ashamed-fearful).

I kept trying to get up. I kept trying to get up as if nothing had happen. I had many changes in areas of my life (attitude-language-body- personality). I was different and it just wasn't apparent. I kept trying to go on; I kept falling down (as Karen and Celtic), I kept trying to go on; get up; regroup, only to fall down over and over again.

Eventually I went to all the necessary places (Church-St. Joseph The Worker-Fr. Paul McQuillen, Mental Health –Algier branch-Dr. Wantpa, Family Services of greater New Orleans- Ginger and Lydia, Y.W.C.A. of Greater L.A.-Compton Ca.- Cynthia, Southern Christian Leadership Conference of Greater L.A.- Rosa Parks A.S.C.C.- Aggy and Stephenie, West Jefferson Medical Center-DR.Shaundra Jones- Lab. Meadowcrest Hospital. I would have tried anything if it would have taken those curses (monkeys) off my back. I would have done anything just to feel better. I didn't ask God Why, I only asked how long?

On Halloween "October99,"After selling my house, I was living at my daughter's house in Algiers Louisiana off the levee. I was home alone, and all of a sudden I could feel myself getting anxious (panicky). I was so anxious that I kept moving from one end of the sofa to the other end and when this didn't work, I went into the bedroom; turned on the television and laid across the bed. In my turmoil, there presented itself a voice, asking me; why don't you take yourself to the levee and walk in the cool water; it will be so refreshing and make you feel so much better. I then became afraid because I knew that

I was in the clutches of the Devil (as Adam-Eve-Jesus). I then became frighten and called on the Lord.

I got on my Knees and prayed and I prayed and I prayed for peace. Not long after I prayed and I prayed for peace (serenity-rest), the Lord appeared and I was able to relax on the couch with the television on, and eventually I just went off to sleep.

I liked the apartments in the complex so much so that I decided to rent me an apartment off the levee to watch the tub boats move up and down the canal. I continue to have the attacks and hear the voices in this new apartment telling me to go to the levee and walk in the cool water, but because I continued to pray; the Lord sent joy to my soul.

My daughter in the complex whom I had lived with eventually bought her a house in Slidell by my other daughter in Slideel. I would visit them often by way of the Twin Span. The voices continued to haunt me when I would travel from Slidell to the West Bank, and the West bank back to Slidell; I decided that I wasn't going to let the Devil take my control.

The Devil (Satan) knew me. The devil knew my thoughts, my likes (dislikes), and that is how he was able to control me. I needed to decided if I was going to heed (hearken) to the voice of the Devil for bad or heed to the voice of God for good, a choice only I could make. In heeding the voice of the Devil, he would automatically make me naked. In heeding the voice of God (Jesus) when He says," come unto Me, all of you who are heavily laden (burdened) and I will give you rest. Take my yoke upon you and learn of Me. For I am meek and lowly in heart; and you shall find rest unto your soul. For My yoke is easy and My burden is light. You will find peace." Matthew 11:28

I took my yoke (burden) to God (Jesus) for good, and through His grace which was sufficient for me, I finally started feeling better. I didn't ask God why. I continued to pray; and then I started to thank him.

I knew that in order for me to continue improving and feel better, I would have to keep doing some of the things that I had been doing already. The reason I would have to continue with the positive was because I knew that my condition was no different from the Alcoholic, the drug abusers, the prostitutes, the sex offenders, etcs, and the only way for me to stay on top of my situation (heal) was to keep walking with God in the straight and narrow and to continue with my positive network. I decided that I had been through hell long enough. I decided that the last days of my life I didn't want to see what someone else had made me. I decided that I didn't want to see all those things of old, all I wanted to see was the Beautiful person that God had made me.

In 2003, I started making progress. I started making plans and really started to get my life together. In 2003, I moved into a nice shot gun house with a shed in the rear. In cleaning this house and sweeping the shed, it was there that I found a big fat rat and heavy powerful dusts. I commended to myself, on how powerful the dust was flying . I remember saying out loud," boy this is some power stuff (shi), and kept on sweeping. I went in the house from the shed with no thoughts to myself in reference to the dust.

At this house there were birds also. At this house these birds lived under the tin roof, and when I would be in the living room watching television, reading and writing with the ceiling fan on, I could swear that something was flying around my face from the fan because there was a small opening in the ceiling. I couldn't see anything, so I just assumed that it was a part of all the craziness (madness). I had been going through.

There came a time when I started itching and scratching; scratching and itching. I started itching in my scalp first and the itch went to my back. My daughter had come to Slidell from California with Celtic for Xmas 2003, and I just assumed that I had gotten these fleas from Celtic as before. I didn't give much notion to the idea that I could have anything else but fleas because, before the holidays was over; we ended up with two dogs instead of one (Celtic from California, a Yorkie and Boss from Slidell, a Maltese. I guess that I just assumed wrong.

One evening while in the living room watching television, my scalp started itching and I scratch it and a bug flew out of my hair. I commended to my son about the bug and he asked me,' mom, why is it that you are the only one who sees these bugs. I didn't get ant sympathy from him.

Some days later, I am in Slidell again, and my back starts to itch again; and I ask my daughter who is a nurse to look at it for me because I was uncomfortable (miserable). My daughter told me that if it's itching that bad then I need to go and see a doctor. I didn't get any sympathy from her either. I decided that if I couldn't get sympathy from my children, why would anyone else listen to me? Just trying to get someone to listen, hear, understand was getting harder and harder to do.

Many bites later, many months later; many months of spending money (buying all kind of products) I just went insane (mad,) waiting and hoping, hoping and waiting, that things would get better. I just lost my pride; I just lost all reasoning, I forgot what others would say and I went to my primary care doctor who didn't waste time getting me out her office; she sent me to a Specialist, she sent me to a dermatology. The Dermatologist started treating me right away.

The Dermatologist started treating me on the same day that I went to see him. He gave me all kinds of information (prescriptions-samples) and told me to return in a couple of days to see if I would need a shot for the itching. I still didn't grasp that the shed and the house (fan) was my biggest problem. I went back into the shed and sweep it out again and took some winter clothes I had put in the shed for storage in the house.

I went back to the doctor's office. I told him that I had gone back in the shed and probably had infected myself again.

I asked him to give me some of the same medicine he had prescribed before and if the medicine didn't give me the results that I needed, I would get a shot for the itching on the next visit.

I ran into two of my first cousins while visiting their brother my cousin in the Hospital. I told them what had been happening to me, and one of my cousins preceded to tell me that some neighbors of hers had gone through the same thing, and I smiled because someone else was going through what I was going through; and then she told me that these neighbors of hers had contacted Scabies, I then frowned.

I threw just about everything I owned (clothes, furniture-etc.) away, and I moved to Slidell. I moved on as I had done in 1999 when I had suffered my first (1st) breakdown.

I moved to Slidell by one of the two daughters I had living in Slidell. I moved to Slidell to isolate myself as my mom had done to isolate herself. I did what I had to do. I did what was familiar to me. I ran as I had done with the abuses. I didn't ask God why? I just continued to pray and ask God how Long?

It was in Slidell that I started to mend. It was in Slidell That I started to regroup again from the breakdown, the scabies. It was in Slidell that I prayed, slowed down; and humbled myself to God. It was because of God (Jesus-the Holy Spirit) and being infected with so many things that I learned how to cry howler, scream, get on my knees to pray; pray and sing and talk to the one who had been my lawyer, pilot, conductor, physician, navigator, friend and advocate. I learned how to pray and talk to the one who had rescued (saved) me.

I went from asking to saying that my affliction was caused by disobedience and I deserved it, to saying that my afflictions was called because I needed to change. I then stopped dealing with the cause of my afflictions and started dealing with the effect of my afflictions, because the effect was doing me in worse then the cause.

My greatest problem was that I had forgot who had been helping (healing) me. I gave credit to all (the doctors, lawyers, Indian chiefs) those I had gone to, and not to the One who had really been helping me. I then started giving credit where credit was due (God-Jesus-the Holy Spirit), and they started sending joy (peace) to my Soul. If it had not been for the Lord on my side where would I have been? I would have still been in prison (naked).I would have still been in prison and the keys would have been still inaccessible. I would have still been in prison and made to pay for all my transgressions; made to pay for all my trust passes. But because I have a High Priest (Advocate) who represented me as my attorney in all my troubles (problems-sins), I now sit back and wonder how I got over. I now sit back and wonder how I got off a prison sentence, because the Devil has been after me (on the prowl), since the beginning of my life causing me headaches (stomach aches), heart aches and pain. The Devil is trying to keep me down in the hole. I didn't ask God (Jesus) Why. I just accepted His help and said thank you.

This is how I got off. This is how I was acquitted due to my Defense Attorney (Jesus) help. I was feeling bad, I was feeling low: I was feeling down and out to the ground and I needed a change. I needed to do something different (radical) because the stressing was causing too much pain; too much suffering; too much hurting when I looked in the mirror. I decided that I had been in pain for most of my life and I didn't want to continue looking in the mirror at all the old abuses, hurts, anguish and imprisonment the flesh man had given me I decided that when I looked in the mirror, all I want to see from now on is the face of God (Jesus); all I want to see is that beautiful woman God had made me.

I prayed and I prayed that Jesus would give me grace. I prayed and I went to Jesus and I told Him that I needed a chance to change the cycle of my life. And then I made another request. I had to make a change (modification) in the request I had made. I had to add another clause to the contract. I asked Jesus to make a detour to pick up some hitch hikers when he came to rescue me. The request I asked Jesus for was for Him to take my children (family) on this journey also. I felt that it wouldn't do me any good for me to change (shift) and they be left behind, because then I would be new (improved) and they would still be looking at the things of old, during the same old things; creating the same old havoc." 1 Cor. 5:7 Holy Bible

I felt that we all had been suffering in Canaan long enough and that it was time for a change, time for us to get away from all the pot holes in the road; away from all my ancient families curses, I didn't ask God why so many curses, I only asked Him how much longer?

I prayed because I was a woman (child-creature) of the dark (night) waiting for my wages, whose life was coming to a swift end. I was as Job who asked the question," Are not our days as those of the hireling? Are not we slaves who longs for the shade, a hireling who waits for his wages. We have been assigned months of misery and troubled nights that has been allotted to us. If we are in bed; we ask when shall we arise? Then the night drags on; and we are filled with restlessness until dawn. Our days are as swifter then a weaver's shuttle that comes to an end without hope. Our life is like the wind and we shall never see happiness again. Job 7:1-4, 6-7 Holy Bible

I didn't phantom that God (Jesus) would have to redeem my life from destruction and crown me with kindness and compassion. Merciful and gracious has been my Father (Jesus), slow to anger and abounding in kindness. Not according to my sins does He deal with me, nor does He deal with me according to my crimes. As far as the East is from the West, and as far as the North is to the South, so far He puts my transgressions from me. As a father has compassion on his children, so does my Father has compassion on those who fear Him." Holy Bible

My father (dad) gave me no compassion. My father had no compassion to give. Because no compassion was given to me, looking in the mirror backwards (negative)has been my only recourse; looking at all those things of old, trying to find some release (relief)." I didn't know that through Christ, (Jesus) all of my old things (mistakes) would pass away and new positives things would be added in its place. I didn't listen to Paul when he said to the Philistines," forget what lies behind, strain forward to what lies ahead in pursuit of that goal." In my misery, I forgot that even though I am going through difficulties other are worst off than me. In my misery, I forgot that even though I am suffering (being held captive) that if I have a hope (dream), a belief, that belief would be the key to my relief. In my misery I forgot that what happens to others (me) shall pass away also. I didn't ask God why? I just went to my Repair man; I just went to my Defense Attorney for my release.

I went to Jesus, the One who is able to replace all my old parts (troubles). I just went to Jesus and told Him about all my troubles and how I am tired of suffering from grief and pain. And that is when everything started to happen that could happen. That is when the cycle change (transition) took effect. Daughter #1, tried to commit Suicide; Daughter #2, almost had a nervous breakdown from the stresses of everyone else problems; Daughter #3, started stressing about her job and problem with her son; Daughter #4, started stressing about her job, and trying to take care of #1 son; Daughter #5, started stressing about her job, school and possibility of an illness, and my son started stressing over his job and life itself. We all started asking the question," what is going on? Daughter #4 said," we must be going through some kind of cycle change because we have never had so many things to happen to all of us at the same time.

I prayed and I prayed. I prayed in season and out of season. The more I seemed to pray (deal with my problems) with God, the worse my problems seemed to get with the Devil.

Eventually I started feeling restless. I started feeling idle; I started feeling a little bit better. I started feeling that I needed to try and go on with my life; and because I was feeling a little better, I started making plans with Ginger (my Therapist) and others to try and move on with my life. I also got in touch with my old Supervisor to see if there was a possibility of me returning to work. Then I got another idea; I then got the idea that I would take some classes at U.N.O.

I only had a few days to register. I had to rush if I was going to get in as a late student. I had some obstacles to face in trying to get in school, but because I prayed, I was successful in enrolling. I was able to enroll, get my classes, and was to start (classes on Monday 8-29-05 of Katrina.

On Saturday before Katrina, while washing dishes and trying to find something to eat; while looking out the kitchen window on a beautiful day, my daughter #4 came into the kitchen to fix herself something to eat and then went into the dining room and between a mouthful of cereal told me to be ready in two (2) hours to leave. I looked at her and asked her to be ready for what? She told me that," she was leaving in two hours and for me to be ready because of the Hurricane. I looked at her strange and asked her what Hurricane are you talking about? She told me Hurricane Katrina. I looked at her and told her that I wasn't going any where's. I also joked and told her that every time a storm (Hurricane) crossed our path, she packs her clothes as if its vacation time again. She asked me mom," haven't you heard that there is a Hurricane out there, and that Hurricane is supposed to be a category 5. I responded and told her no, and that I have had enough of running from Hurricanes (Ivan); I have had enough of packing, locking the house down; traffic and driving. I told her that I felt that I was going to be alright. I told her and the others that I spoke to later," that I had a belief (faith) that I would be alright and that I wasn't going to do as Peter when he had asked Jesus if it was alright for him to walk toward Him on the water; and how Jesus told Peter to come; and how Peter leaped overboard and walked toward Jesus on the water; but when he saw how terrible the storm was he became frighten because of lost of faith, and almost drowned. All or my children (grandsons) in Louisiana fled the State because of the Hurricane.

At (around) ten p.m., I decided to prepare myself for sleep because all lines of communication had started to cut off. In the house on the second floor by the bathroom is where I bunkered down. I had already gutted closets in the house and put survival items in the closets in case I would have to flee from room to room. I had candles, flash lights, water, radio, batteries, food, and etc, just in case I would have need of these items. I especially had God (Jesus), a Bible, a cross, a clock with the picture of Jesus, a candle with the picture of Jesus, and before I went off to sleep I prayed for all of us, those who left and those who stayed. I had a faith: I had a belief that we were all going to be alright. I went down stairs and turned off the electricity control box, and then I went back upstairs to fall asleep.

I went to sleep; Boss went to sleep at approximately ten (10) p.m.). I don't know what Boss heard during the night because he isn't saying. I didn't hear anything again until the following morning (Aug. 29, 2005). Boss and I woke up around the time we usually get up. And that is when it hit me that we had survived a Hurricane .I thought as before that the Hurricane had probably turned and went in another direction. It was dark outside, the wind was blowing; the rain was falling and there was plenty noise to be heard. I looked out the window and it was still early morning. I peeped out the door and it was just as dark out there. I looked out the door; I looked at Boss, and told him that he was on his own. I shut the door and we went back upstairs, blew out the candle, and went back to sleep as I usually do when there is a Hurricane.

I don't know till this day when the storm passed. The eye did pass and because the Lord had put me in a deep sleep (as Adam) so I wouldn't hear or see anything of the storm; and because He had put a hedge around me, I didn't witness to much of what had happened with the storm.

I went back to sleep thanking God (Jesus) for His goodness. I went back to sleep thanking God for His mercy as I had often done before. I went to sleep with the idea that I would either be on this side of the earth when the storm was over or I would have gone to the other side with Jesus; either side that I be on would be alright with me because it would be the will of God. I didn't ask God why? I just said thank you.

The next time that I woke up from sleep, the outside wasn't as dark; it was much clearer this time around. I peeped out the door cautiously and I could see that a lot of trees had fallen for days. I saw the giant (big) pine tree which sets in front of my daughter's house that we both loved was now lying across the yard. And the beauty (blessing) of God's Glory is that we had been warned that that tree would fall one day in my daughter's house, and instead of going in the direction that it was predicted to fall in, it went the opposite way.

Later I saw many trees in the back yard had fallen and a few sidings from the house were missing. Then I surveyed the neighbor's houses. The house to the left of my daughter's house had plenty damage, while the neighbor to the right had hardly no damage. Several houses in the surrounding area had trees that had fallen in their roofs (houses); shingles, siding and fence problems, while some didn't have any problems at all. I looked at all the damage that had occurred and I said to God," Yes Lord, You sure have been busy out here; and I wondered how the house on the left had sustained a lot of damage and the house on the right had sustained hardly any damage at all.

When looking at the damage to my daughter's house and looking at the damage to her neighbor's houses, I then thought of how my daughter's would ask if it weren't time for me to go on vacation because of something I would have said or done; I then smiled and asked the Lord, Hey is this all the damage you are going to do to this house after all the times they have sent me on vacation. You must be going to send something else? You must be going to let something else happen? And before I could finish getting the words out of my mouth, my daughter's big giant Chimney from her fire place felled with a big (loud) bang. I then smiled.

I had no idea as to what was happening in other parts of Slidell or anywhere else for that matter because my radio was acting up. I had no idea that my children thought that I was dead for three days because the radio announcement (communication- information) had said that Slidell was gone, and the Twin span was gone also. I didn't realize that New Orleans my city ; New Orleans my habitat, New Orleans my friend had slipped away; I didn't realize that New Orleans my city: New Orleans my Habitat, New Orleans my friend had passed away; I didn't realize that New Orleans my city; New Orleans my Habitat, New Orleans my friend had now gone on. The reality of New Orleans death has now set in; the reality that there will be no more trips to New Orleans has now set in. the reality that there will be no more calls to New Orleans to tell her that I love her has now set in, the reality has now set in that New Orleans my beloved City has moved on.

The day after New Orleans died Boss and I are home alone. We are home alone and I am down and out thinking about New Orleans (family and friends). We are home alone and I am down and out thinking about New Orleans; her illness and her death. We are home alone and I am down and out thinking about how life is unfair; and how life took the children as well as the parents. I am so engrossed in my thinking that suddenly tears starts to flow from my eyes and there is no one shoulder to lay my head; I am so engrossed in my thoughts and tears and there is no one to talk to, to tell them what and how I am feeling about New Orleans demise, and just as the lightening begins to flash; and just as the thunder begins to roar, then there is this impregnable (strong) voice which say's," I do not slumber nor do I sleep, I have not caused the flood waters to flow, but yes I have caused the Hurricane to roar, for My benefit (Glory); for your benefit, just as I did when I brought you through the Red Sea; just as I did when I brought you through the Jordan River; Just as I did when I put you to sleep and sheltered you from the storm. I have caused the Hurricane to happen and let the flood waters of the flesh (man) to flow, not just for the benefit of the Gulf Coast, but for the benefit of the whole world (nation). I have let this disaster happen to see what My people would do in their time of troubles; to see what they would do when I hid My face from them; to see what they would do when they didn't have Me to pull them from the waters (Katrina -flood-Rita).

All of my children (family) are now scattered in different parts of the country (as in Towel of Babel). My daughter who I had been living with has now taken a new job, sold her house, bought another house, and have now moved on. I then had a problem. I had a problem because all of my children had benefited from the cycle change (blessing). I then had a problem because all of my children had landed some where's positive (promising) except me. I thought! I didn't ask God why. I asked where to?

I ended up putting my tail between my legs and headed to California. My daughter and my son-in-law made me welcome; they satisfied me. I couldn't understand God's motives; I couldn't understand God's reason for sending me to live with my daughter (son-in-law) who had on many instances already sheltered homeless individuals from theirs storms (situations).

I couldn't understand how God answered my pray for my children but hadn't answered my prayer for me. And then I started thinking about a prayer I had sent up to my Father God-Jesus) before leaving for California. I then remembered while Traveling to Church, how I would see all the devastation of Gentily; all the devastation of the nineth (9th) ward; All the devastation of the seventh (7th) ward; all the devastation of St. Bernard Parish; all the devastation of Lakeview; all the devastation of the eight (8th) ward; all the devastation of Jefferson Parish, and Orleans Parish (Kenner); and St Tammany Parish (Slidell), and how I told the Lord that It had been a mighty long journey and I had struggle alone the way; it has been a long ride and I was tired.

I also told Him, how it had been a long voyage and that I needed Him to send me a chauffer (train-bus-plane) to take me somewhere where it is quiet so that I could get me some rest from everyone and everything. I told Him that I was tired and that I just felt as though I couldn't go on. And that is when He told me, "one more day, one more step; I'm preparing you for myself. When you can't hear my voice, please trust my plan, I am the Lord; I see and hear and yes I understand." Smokey N.

I was put on a train and sent to Inglewood California. I later realized that my problem was the fact that I was in the robust (fortified-powerful) city of California. My problem was that I was used to New Orleans (Marrero-Slidell). California for me is a place to visit (enjoy)' not a place to live. I started questioning God often about me living in California. I ask God why? I asked God how long? I begged Him to get me out of California; and then I had to admonish (caution) myself for having these thoughts because there are so many others who didn't have a California to flee (runoff) to. I realized then that I had a life of ease; I had been blessed often even with all the curses (craziness). I had someone to go to and live with in my time of despair (need), while there were many families (friends) and others who had no one to rely on they thought! They had God (Jesus) to rely on.

There were also many friends (family) who had made me realize before Katrina and after Katrina that I had been treated different (better). They also told me that I had been treated better than my sister. I started feeling faulty (unfavorable-evil-sinful-corrupted-tainted-naked) when I was told that I had been treated better. I started thinking that maybe I had been unappreciative. I started thinking that I had been inconsiderable (too big for myself). The last straw came when I had called a friend of mines to tell him Happy Birthday, and before I could get off the phone; he went on to tell me how I had been treated better (different) from my sister. I wonder if my sister called him and wished him Happy Birthday. Ha, ha, ha.

I let them weigh me down with guilt. I let them make me feel bad, and then I started thinking about my life; my sister life, and then I started thinking about how different my sister and I accepted our lives (fate-Being). I started thinking about how many years ago , there were two (2) sisters, born to the same father and mother; many years ago these two sisters were abandon by their father when one was three (3) months old, and the other not born yet; many years ago these two sisters grandfather (grandmother) died before they were five (5) years old. Many years ago these two sisters mother died when one was five (5) years old and the other was four (4) years old. Many years ago these two sisters were abused (made naked-undressed, ashamed)by their new parents whose care they were placed in by God; Many years ago these two sisters were both in prison (Egypt) and escaped by way of the Red Sea. Many years ago these two sisters wandered forty (40) years in the wilderness so that God could humble them; Many years ago these two sisters escaped the wilderness by way of the Jordan River and finally entered into Canaan and did what they wanted to do instead of what God wanted them to do. They rejected God's orders to rid themselves of the inhabitants of the land. They started doing some of the things (sins) that the old inhabitants were doing. They started worshipping idol gods and marrying of the inhabitants. They started acting just like them and doing the opposite of what God wanted for them. They did what Satan wanted. They let him take their control." Joshua exhorted (Implored) my sister and me to be strong and courageous; to keep God's commandments; to love the Lord, and neither marry among or cleave unto the remnants of the Canaanites who remained in the land. We were warned that if we served other gods, we would be cursed and dispossessed." Joshua 23:1-16

"Worshiping false gods only brought severe judgment upon us (Israelites-Gentiles-my sister and myself), but in the end, we shall be reconciled to our Father (God) and be His people." Hebrew 2:1-23

"Joshua recites how the Lord led us out from captivity. He told us to choose God and to serve Him only." Joshua 24:1-33

These two sisters were as the seven (7) ward in New Orleans, One area was rich (St. Augustine School- St Peter Claver-Corpus Christi, while the other area was poor (St Raymond Church- Nelson-Phillip School); these two sisters were as Celtic and Boss, two pedigreed dogs (two cousins) for two different sisters. Celtic is the inside dog who walks in front; gets a lot of attention and always complaint , while Boss is the outside dog who walks behind, gets less attention and never complaints. These two sisters are like Saul and David. Saul is made King by God (who is our King of Kings) because this is what the people wanted. Then Saul is rejected by God because of sin and David is then chosen to be king; and Saul sets out to kill David because of jealousy. I Samuel 8:1-22, 10:1-3, 13:1-23 -These two sisters are as the Mayor of Slidell and the Mayor New Orleans; The Mayor of New Orleans C. Ray Nagin is black and the Mayor of Slidell is White.

The Mayor of New Orleans had plenty damage (devastation-destruction) from Hurricane Katrina (Rita-the flood) and the Mayor of Slidell had less damage; The city of New Orleans received less Support after the Flood (Hurricanes) The city of Slidell received much Support after the Hurricane (flood). Was God fair to my sister?

Many felt that life had treated me better (preferable) than my sister. Do God judge and make distinction among His Children? Is everyone treated equally? Is everyone really treated the same? Who are the Israelites to whom pertain the adoption and the glory; and the covenant; and the given of the Law, and the service of God and the promise. Whose are the Father's and whom as concerning the flesh Christ came, who is over all, God blessed forever. Amen not as though the world God has taken no effect, for they are all not Israel which are Israel. Neither, because they are seeds of Abraham are they all His children. That is," they which are children of the flesh, these are not children of God, but the children of the promise to be counted for the seed. For this is the word of the Promise," At a specific time I will come, and Sara shall have a son, and not only this, but When Rebecca had also conceived by one, even by our Father Isaac: for the children being not yet born, neither having good or evil, that the purpose of God according to the election might stand; not of works, but of Him that called. It was said unto her, the elder shall serve the younger. As it is written: Jacob have I loved, but Esau have I hated. What shall we say then? Is there Unrighteousness with God? God forbid. For God said to Moses," I will have mercy on whom I will have mercy and I will have compassion on whom I will have compassion. So then, it is not of him that will it, nor of him that run it, but of God that shows mercy. Roman 9: 1-33 For the Scripture said unto Pharaoh, even for this purpose have I raised thee up, that I might show My power in thee, and that My name might be declared through all the earth. Therefore has He mercy on whom He will have mercy and whom He will harden. Thou will say then unto Me, why does He yet find faith? For who hast resisted His will? Nay, but who of man; who art thou that repliest against God? Shall the things formed say to Him that formed it," Why hast thou made me thus? Has not the potter power over the clay of the same lump to make one vessel unto honor, and another dishonor. What if God, willing to show His wrath, and to make His power known, endures with much long suffering the vessels of wrath fitted to destruction; and that He might make known the riches of His glory on the vessel of mercy, which He had before prepared unto; even us, whom He has called, not of the Jews only, but also of the Gentles," Roman 9:1-13

Everyone said that life treated me better, but no one came to rescue her, no one came to rescue me, and because no one came to save (rescue) us we didn't have the wisdom that founded the earth nor the understanding that established the Heaven. We didn't have the knowledge that broke up the depths or the clouds that drop the dew. We let them depart from our eyes and didn't keep sound wisdom and discretion, so that they might be life unto our soul, and grace to our neck. We didn't walk in safety and our feet did stumble because no one came for us, no one rescued us.

It was in California that the Cycle (shift) change did start to take effect even though I didn't realize it. In California, not only did I go to Church, but I walked often; found three (3) different therapists (Y.W.C.A.-Rosa Parks etc.), and called on Ginger (Family Service of Greater New Orleans) to get her views on my situations.

Because I didn't know my way around, I started catching the bus. I started catching the bus to learn my way around; and found many nice individuals (Hispanics- blacks- whites-etc) who were in worse predicaments then I was. I started walking, talking and riding with these different individuals (homeless) and found out that they were no different from me, down to earth).They (like me) didn't have much money; they had much love, so they didn't have anything to lose.

It was in California that I started to relax; a relaxation that I had never had before. I found in California that the only one I had to be accountable to is God. The only one I have to look up to is God (Jesus) because He alone holds my destiny in His hands. I also was told by a co-walker (Bob) to stop trying to change others, because the only one I can change is me.

I started feeling that the cycle change was working. I then realize in California that I was free; that my children (grandchildren) was free thanks to God (Hurricane Katrina-the flood) and if we go back to our old ways of life (habits-prison), it would be because of our choices and not because of the choices of others.

My life then went into reverse, my life then started going back in time. Many told me that I shouldn't be looking backwards; many told me looking backward would only make matters worse (make me naked).

I then started reliving these things of old. I then started having P.T.S.D. (flashes-disassociation-being trigger); I then started screaming, howling and kicking in my sleep all over again, but it is funny now; it is funny now because as I am going (looking) backwards in time these things of old are being erased from my memory bank, and the beauty (blessing) of my remembering these things of old, I started remembering how it was God (Jesus) who carried (rescued) me when I was drowning from the weight of my imprisonment. I saw how they rescued (saved) me from all of my frights and fears; how they saved me before the Hurricane; during the Hurricane; and after the Hurricane; how they saved me from the bugs, and nervous breakdown; how they saved me from toxicemia when my son was born; how they saved me from drowning when I was in a car accident and my car went into a ditch; how they saved me when I lost a lot of blood due to an abortion; how they saved me from the abuses (physical-mental-verbal-sexually; how they saved me when my father left; how they saved me when my grandfather (grandmother) died; how they saved me when my mother died. I saw how they saved me, how they rescued me; how they carried me, I finally opened my eyes and now I can see; I finally opened my eyes and saw God my President; God my King; God my Savior. I finally opened my eyes and saw Jesus the Healer; I finally saw Jesus the One who has cured all of my aches and pain.

Who is this Jesus? Where did He come from? Why do we have to go to Him instead of God? Jesus is the son of God; the son of David; the son Abraham (Isaac and Jacob) the kingly ancestors who lived about a thousand years after Abraham. While the genealogy shows the continuity of Gods providential plan for Abraham on discontinuity o f God's plan from Abraham on, discontinuity also present in the women Tamar, Rehab, Ruth and the wife of Uriah (Bathesheba) who bore their sons through unions that were in varying degrees strange and unexpected. These irregularities culminate in the supreme "irregularity" of the Messiah's birth of a virgin mother; the age of fulfillment is inaugurated by a creative act of God. "This is how the birth of Jesus Christ came about: His mother Mary was pledged to be married to Joseph, but before they could come together, she was found with child through the Holy Spirit." Matthew 1:1-18; Because Joseph her husband was a righteous man and did not want to expose her to public disgrace; he had in mind to divorce her quietly." Matthew 1:19 Holy Bible 'Behold a virgin shall be with child and shall bring forth a son and they shall call His name Emmanuel, for in Him, God is with us. The announcement of the birth of this new born King of the Jews greatly troubled not only Herod but all of Jerusalem, yet the Gentiles Magi are overjoyed to find Him and offer Him homage and their gifts, thus His ultimate rejection by the mass of His own people and the acceptance by the Gentile nation is foreshadowed; He Must be taken into Egypt to escape the murderous plan of Herod." Matthew 2:13

Holy Bible," By His sojourn there and His subsequent return after the King's death, He relives the subsequent experience of Israel; "The word of the Lord spoken through Hosea," Out of Egypt I called My Son." Matthew 2:15,"If Israel was the Son of God, Jesus is so in a way far surpassing the dignity of that nation; as is His marvelous birth, and the unfolding of His History. Matthew 3:17 4:1-11 11:27 14:33 Holy Bible

Back in the land of Israel He must be taken to Nazareth in Galilee because of the danger to His life in Judea where Herod's son Archelaus is now ruling." Matthew 22:23 The suffering of Jesus in the infancy narrative anticipated those of His passion and His life is spared of the danger, it is because His destiny is finally to give it on the cross as a ransom for many; Even as the son of Man came not to be ministered unto, but to minister (serve) and give His life." John the Baptist preached in the wilderness of Judea, saying, "repent for the Kingdom of God is at hand. For this is He that was spoken of by the prophet Esaias, saying, voice of one crying in the wilderness, prepare ye the way of the Lord, make His path straight." Then there's the Baptism of Jesus that culminates in God's proclaiming Him as His beloved Son. The central message of Jesus preaching is the coming of the Kingdom of Heaven is at hand and the need for Repentance, a complete change of heart and conduct on the part of those who are to receive this great gift of God. Jesus fame spreads to all of Syria, and brought Him all who were sick with various diseases and racked with pain; those who are possessed, lunatics and paralytics and He cured them all. Great crowds from Galilee, Decropolis, Jerasalem, and from beyond the Jordon followed Him. There were many things He taught them also; He taught the Beatitude, The Similes of salt and light: the teaching of the Law; the teaching of anger, adultery, divorce, oaths, retaliation, fasting, Treasures stored up in Heaven, the light of the body, God and money, dependence on God, judging of others, pearls and the swine etc. Jesus surpasses Himself because He was also given the power to raise individuals from the grave, including Lazarus His friend. He also taught that our living (our neighbors-children must be helped. When the disciples tried to prevent the children from coming to Jesus, Jesus rebuked them saying," Let the children come to Me, and do not hinder them, for it is to just such as these that the Kingdom belongs. By this he meant that to obtain Heaven His disciples (we) must become like a child in their humility and simplicity, and in their belief and trust in God. After the children had gathered around Him, Jesus laid His hand upon them and blessed them." Mark 10:13-16

What must we do to be saved? One of the most solemn and meaningful events in the entire life of Jesus was the Last Supper. During the last meal of Jesus and His Disciples, Jesus reclined at the table with the twelve disciples (apostles) and spoke of His approaching betrayal by one of those present. He further indicated that the events of the betrayal, arrest, conviction and execution has been the subject of divinely inspired prophesies and all that which was to follow was the fulfillment of the will of God. After the Pascal Supper, Jesus instituted the Holy Eucharist; The Sacrament and Sacrifice of His Body and His Blood. Taking a loaf of unleavened bread and breaking it into portions for each one of those present; He blessed it and gave it to His disciples saying," take this and eat, this is my body; He then took the cup, gave thanks and gave it to them and said," all of you must drink from it; for this is the blood, the blood of the everlasting Covenant to be poured out in behalf of many for the forgiveness of sins. He then asked those present to continue to carry out this same ordinance of bread and wine in commemoration of His own bloody Sacrifice on the Cross for the sins of all mankind which was soon to transpire. Holy Bible

After supper, Jesus took Peter, James, and John along with Him to the garden of Gethsemane. Inside He knelt down a short distance apart from the others and began to pray. Jesus was sad and sorely troubled, having a divine knowledge of His sufferering and Crucifixation to come. Sweating drops of blood in His agony, He pleaded with His Heavenly Father that He might be spared this ordeal, yet He was resigned to accept His Father's will saying," My Father if it is possible, let this Cup Pass by Me." Still Lord let it be as You would have it and not as I would have it." Jesus was found guilty of a crime He didn't commit. Jesus was found guilty of Blasphemy by the Jewish Sanhedrin, and His punishment of death was demanded by the clamoring crowd. After prolong efforts to evade the Judgment, which was to be fulfilled. Pilate finally yielded to the Jewish authorities (yielded to the pressure like Lynndie), and the demands of the Mob and issued the order that Jesus was to be Crucified on the Cross. Matthew 27:33-36

The will of God is a lonely one for those who are called. It is lonely because not many will want to do His will but their will. They will want the crown but not the cross. They will have a hard concept that the crown is not given unless the cross is given. In applying for the Job, those who apply must remember that the Son of God (Jesus) didn't have a bed to sleep on and the conditions that He live in wasn't perfect." And when they had platted a crown of thorns, they put it on His head and a reed in His right hand and they bowed and kneeled before Him, and mocked Him saying," Hail, King of the Jews; and they spit on Him, and took the reed and smote Him on the head; and after that they took His robe off Him and put His raiment on Him, and led Him away to be crucified. Matthew 27:29-31

"And they crucified Him, and parted His garments, casting lots that it might be fulfilled which was spoken by the prophets. They parted His garments among themselves and upon His vesture did they cast lots. Then from the sixth (6th) hour there was darkness over the land unto the ninth (9th) hour; and about the ninth (9th) hour Jesus cried out with a loud voice, saying, Eli, Eli, lama sabachthan? That is to say," My God, My God, why has thou Forsaken (Abandon) Me?

Many who heard Jesus said, "let us see whether Elias will come and save Him."

For a good number of years, I cried out silently for my father to come and rescue me. For many years I cried out in a silent voice, "My father, my father, why hast thou forsaken (Abandon) me. He came back many years later, but wasn't able to rescue (help) me because I was too far gone. God, my Father, will have to send a Redeemer (Jesus) to save me from the storms (trials). God will have to send Jesus to rescue me from the grave.

"Jesus when he had cried again with a loud voice yielded up the ghost and died. And behold the veil of the temple was rent in twain from the top to the bottom; and the earth did quake and the rocks rent; and the graves were opened; and many bodies of the saints which slept arose; and came out of the grave after Jesus Resurrection, and went into the Holy city, and appeared to many. Matthew 27:1-66, so that the Scripture would be fulfilled".

"When Christ died on the Cross there was great mourning among the people who had followed Him. Among them were Mary Magdalene and Mary the mother of James and John. They were joined by Joseph of Arimathea who was also a disciple of Christ. He had gone to Pilate to get permission to take down the body of Christ." Mark 15:42-47

In mourning the death of Jesus, and when mourning the death of a love one (Karen- New Orleans); when we mourn these events we must remember that death is the will of God due to Adam. When we mourn these happy events hopefully we are mourning them with hope, joy, and love in our heart, because Jesus made it possible for us have peace.

"After the Resurrection, because of love, joy, and peace, Jesus ate with His Apostles and led them to mount Olive where

He continued to walk and talk with them. Finally He lifted up His hands and blessed them and as He did this, He was lifted up to Heaven before their eyes, and a cloud took Him out of their sight. Enraptured, the Apostles fell down on their knees; worshiped Him, and then they returned to Jerusalem with great joy in their heart." Luke 24:36-51

God sent His Son for a plan and a purpose. God sent Katrina for a plan and purpose also. Jesus (Hurricane Katrina-the flood) came because we had stepped out of the safety net of God. Jesus (Hurricane Katrina The flood) came because we had forged ahead and forgot to take the helpless; forgot to take the homeless; forgot to take the hopeless alone with us as God had required. Jesus came for Redemption and Repentance. Jesus (Hurricane Katrina-the flood) was sent by God as another chance for us to go forward; as another chance to move with Christ, as another chance to see what we will do.

God knew of our old habits of conforming to the norm. He knew of our habit of going back to what we are familiar with, and so He did to us what He did to the people of time past. He did to us what He did to the people of Noah's time; He spread us all over the world as a new start and to prevent us from becoming naked; and to prevent us from sinning, Jesus came for Accountability.

With accountability, God has decided that He is going to make us pay for our actions. Before the Hurricane (flood) we did everything unimaginable to disrespect God and were able to get away with these sins because of Jesus the Redeemer who died for us. And now after the flood God has deemed it necessary to hold us accountable for our actions (sins). Jude ," the servant of Jesus Christ and brother of James said to them that are sanctified by God the Father and preserved in Jesus Christ,' Mercy unto you, and peace, and love be multiplied. Beloved, when I gave all diligence to write unto you of the common salvation, it was needed for me to write unto you and exhort you that you should earnestly contend for the faith which was once delivered unto the saints. For there were certain men whose condemnation was written long ago have secretly slipped in among us. They are godly men who change the grace of our God into a license for immorality and deny Jesus Christ our only Sovereign and Lord. Though we already know this that the Lord delivered His people out of Egypt, but later those who did not believe; and the angels who did not keep their position of authority but abandoned their own home; These He kept in darkness, bound with everlasting chains for judgment on the great day. In similar ways, Sodom and Gomorrah and the surrounding towns gave themselves up to Sexual immorality and perversion. He serve as an example of those who suffer the punishment of eternal fire. In the same way, these dreamers pollute their own bodies, reject authority and slander celestial beings. But even the archangel Michael, when he was disputing with the devil about the body of Moses, did not dare to bring slanderous against him, but said," the Lord rebuke you. Yet these men speak abusively against whatever they do not understand; and what things they do understand by instinct, like unreasoning animals; these are the things that destroys them. Woe to them that has the understanding of Cain. Jude 1:1-11

The Question to be asked now is," will the plan (accountability plan) work? Not even Jesus may be able to solve the problem of sin, because it lives deep down inside our heart.

God honored the people of the Gulf Coast, He honored the Gulf Coast (New Orleans) by giving us a chance to change the course of History; He honored us by giving us a chance to change the course of many years past; He honored us by letting us change a wrong into a right. We can now honor Him by making a cycle change, by shifting forward rather than shifting backwards.

The Gulf coast is defunct now, because of Hurricane Katrina (Rita-the flood); the Gulf Coast is defunct because many have lost their lives, homes, jobs, businesses, livelihood, and the necessary (heart) to go on in the aftermath of the storm. We have resorted to going backward as the Israelite rather then finishing the race with God (Jesus). We did the ultimate failure by not calling on God (Jesus) in our time of distress (despair); we did the ultimate disrespect when we called on the Government (the natural), as our Savior, and neglected to acknowledge God (Jesus) as our Lord and Savior who is able to do all things. We failed to realize that the battle was not our, that the battle was the Lord's. We failed to realize that Katrina (Rita-the flood) was meant as a cleaning; as a purging; as a time of renewal for all of us. God didn't discriminate with His judgment with the Hurricane (Gulf Coast) and He won't discriminate with His judgment on our leaders (our President, Preachers, Priests, Teachers etc), when they fail to instruct His children in the way to go. Malachi says," If you will not listen and if you will not set your heart to honor my name says the Lord Almighty," I will sent a curse upon you, and I will curse your children (blessings). You have turned aside from My ways and have caused many to falter by your instructions. You have made me void the covenant of the Levi's says the Lord of Host. I have thereby made you contemptible and base before all the people; since you do not keep My ways, but shows partiality in your decisions. Have we not all one Father? Did not one God create us all? Why do you profane the covenant of our Father by breaking Faith with another? Malachi 1-14, 2-26, 8-10 Sunday Missal

Right now we are all under a curse because of our corruptible ways (past), and in order for us to find the peace that surpasses all understanding, we will have to go back to the original plan of God before Adam. We will have to go back to the Beginning (Bible) which says," In you oh Lord, I have found peace. Lord my heart is not proud; my eyes are not hearty. I busy myself not with great things or with things too sublime for me. Oh Israel (Gulf Coast-New Orleans), renew your Faith (hope) in the Lord both now and forever. Psalm 131 Sunday Missal

If we the Gulf Coast (nation) would only heed to the words of the Father (God) and not withdraw (stray) from Him, we then can continue to be considered His chosen Ones moving into the Promise Land." A vine from Egypt you transplanted. You drove away the nations and planted them. You put forth it's foliage to the sea, and it shoots as far as the river. Why have you broken its walls, that every passerby plucks its fruits; the boars from the forest lays it waste on it; and the beast of the field feeds on it? Once again, o Lord of host look down from heaven and see me; take care of this vine and protect what your right hand has planted; whom your right hand has made strong, that we will no more withdraw from You. Father," Give us a new life, and we will call upon Your name. O Lord of host, please renew us (your people); and let Your face shine upon us, so that we shall be saved and never be made naked again." Sunday Missal.

In order for us to find grace, in order for us to find mercy, in order for the Lord face to shine upon us, we will have to look forward; we will have to look ahead and stop looking backward (for the things of old); stop looking for the Garden of Eden; stop looking for the old Ark of Noah; stop looking for Sodom and Gomorrah; stop looking for Egypt; stop looking for Canaan; stop looking for Katrina, we are going to stop looking for those things because the only thing these things will do for us is bring us back to a place where we don't want to go. We will have to do what Paul told the Philistines to do," He told them to Pray to our Father for all of our needs. He will guard over us. Discern what is true, noble, good and pure, loved, and honored; virtuous or worthy of praise. God's peace will then be on us." Phil. 4:6-9   Brother and sisters have no anxiety at all, but in everything by prayer and petition; with thanks make your request known in God. Then the Peace of God that surpasses all understanding will guard your hearts and mind in Jesus Christ. Finally, brothers and sisters whatever is just; whatever is pure; whatever is gracious; if there is any excellence and if there is anything worthy of praise, think about these things. Keep on doing what you have learned, receive, heard and seen in Me (God), then the   God   of Peace will be with you always.   Phil 4:6-9   Sunday Missal

And the question now is," Why are we suffering? We are Suffering now because we didn't keep our eyes on the prize (God-Jesus). We are suffering now because we failed to live as if today will be our last day; we are suffering because we failed to do God's will, we did the flesh will. And in order to make this wrong a right, we will have to walk in the straight and narrow, and go humbly into He throne of grace and admit to our trespasses through Jesus Christ and ask Him to forgive us. We will have to follow His laws and His decrees and His Commandments; and then and only then He may give us another "Chance" to Change a wrong into a right in Spite of Our Obstacles, and maybe He'll help us Weather the Storms.

Isaiah speaks Messianically of the Messiah," The Lord hath given me the tongue of the learned, so that I shall know how to speak a word in season to him that is weary; he wakes up morning by morning, he awake my ear to hear as the learned. The Lord God hath opened my ear, and I was not rebellious, neither did I turn my back. I gave my back to the smiters, and my cheeks to them that plucked off my hair. I hid my face from shame and spitting. For the Lord God will help me, therefore shall I not be conformed; therefore have I set my face like a flint, and know that I shall not be ashamed (naked). He is near and justified me who will contend with me? Let him come near me. Behold the Lord will help me; who is he that shall condemn me? Lo! They all shall wax old as a garment; the moth shall eat them up. Who is among you that fear the Lord, that obeys the voice of His servant; that walks in darkness, and has no light? Let him trust in the name of the Lord and stay upon His God. Behold all of you that kindle a fire; that compass yourselves about with sparks, walks in the light of your fire and in the sparks that you have kindled. This shall you have of my hand; you shall lie down in sorrow." Isaiah (Holy Bible)

In making these things right, we need to ask ourselves the question, did we help anyone lately instead of giving lip service and worrying about self? Did we help anyone like Oprah winfrey and Bill gates did? Did we help Ieone Wilson when she lost eleven members of her family all at the same time like Derrick Shepherd , Sheriff Harry Lee, Davis Mortuary; St. Joseph The Worker Catholic Church (Fr. Paull McQuillen , Bishop Paul Morton, Bishop Innis Antoine etc? Did we help the victims of the World Trade Center (N.Y.); Did we help any of the victims of Hurricane Katrina (flood-Rita) Did you help the two abused sisters (brother); Did we help the homeless (hungry); did we step up to the place for the Feed The Children Program, etc, for when the Son of God comes in His Glory and all the Angels with Him, He (Jesus) will sit on His throne in Heavenly Glory. All the nation (Gulf Coast) will be gathered before Him, and He will separate the people from another as a Shepherd separates a sheep from a goat. He will put the sheep on the right and the goats on the left. Then the King (Jesus) will say to those on His right, come, you who are blessed by My Father; take your inheritance; for the Kingdom has been prepared for you since the creation of the world. For when I was hungry you gave me something to eat; when I was thirsty you gave something to drink; when I was a stranger you invited me in; when I needed clothes you clothed me, and when I was sick (in Prison), you visited me. And the King will say," I tell you the truth, what ever you did to the least of these children of mines, you did unto Me. Then He will say to those on the left, Depart, from me, you who are cursed into the eternal fire prepared for the devil and his angels. For when I was hungry you gave me nothing to eat; when I was thirsty, you gave me nothing to drink; when I was a stranger; you didn't invite me in; when I needed clothes; you clothed me not; when I was sick (in prison) you did not visit me. They will also answer, Lord," when did we see you hungry, or thirsty, or a stranger, or needing clothes, or sick, or in prison, and did not help you? Then the Lord will reply," I tell you the truth, what you did not do for the least of these children, you did not for Me (Jesus). Then they will go away to their eternal punishment, but the righteous will go to eternal life. Matthew 25:31-46

We as a nation will have to do away with the notion that what applies to others (Whites-Black-Jews-Hispanics-Chinese-Japanese-Democrats-Republicans-Conservatives-Baptist-Catholic-Methodist-etc; do not apply to us. Whatever judgment applies to one; applies to all, are there but One God; are there but One Jesus; Are there but One Holy Spirit; wasn't there but One Adam. We all are under One Body, One God (Jesus), created in the image of that One God. A sin, is a sin, is a sin, no matter who is committing that sin. We all have to do the Will of God, no matter who we are.

We All Are Going To Be Held Accountable For What We Do Now; Just Look At Iraq; Just Look At New Orleans; Just look at all murders; Just Look At All The Abuses (Physical-Mental-Verbal-Sexual); Just Look At All The Things we are doing that is not of God. We all (The Nation-My Sister, Brother And Myself) will have to make God (Jesus) our President, King, Savior and Father.